The systemic Integrative Thinking Approach to Problem Solving Vol: I

It's Application in Healthcare
OBESITY:
Prevention & Management

Kwasi Yeboah-Afihene

A DISCLAIMER

The information in this book in its entirety is not a medical advice, and no one should use it to either diagnose any health indication or self medicate. My advice to you thought is that, if anyone fells he has a need for any medical attention related to his or her health in any form, should contact his or her physician, or any physician if he or she does not have one already. It is very risky to your health for picking any information anywhere, and act on it to self medicate without the appropriate consultation of a respective qualified and certified healthcare practitioner.

Also the various phenomena being described regarding OBESITY and related issues in this book, are DEEMED UNIVERSAL. Specific Examples or samples are used to describe them not with the intent of any specificity to any individual or systems or subsystems. As broad as I will attempt to describe them, it is a human phenomenon universal to our common humanity, and global landscape. Its applications should be abstracted and applied with individual culturally appropriate nuances. [THANKS, AUTHOR]

Copyright © 2014 by **Kwasi Yeboah-Afihene**

Library of Congress Control Number: Pending

ISBN-13: 978-1497400009
ISBN-10:1497400007

All rights reserved. No part of this book may be reproduced or transmitted in any form or by any means, electronic or mechanical, including photocopying, recording, or by any information storage and retrieval system, without permission in writing from the copyright owner.

This book was printed in the United States of America.

Author's contact details:

Kwasi_afihene@yahoo.com
[Also on LinkedIn and Facebook]

Dedication:

This book is dedicated to my HEROS in Health and Wellness, including OBSEITY and related health complications, nationally and globally. Though they are many, I will mention a few who has made personal and group, significant strides which are worth noticing, though everyone's, big or small contribution helped, or is helping turn the flying wheel. I believe it will accelerate in momentum pretty soon.

They are:

>Mrs. Michel Obama *(First Lady)*
>
>Mr. Michel Bloomberg *(Former NY Mayor)*
>
>Mr. and Mrs. William Gates
>
>Mr. Warren Buffet

Honorable President William J. Clinton

Mrs. Hilary Clinton *(Former First Lady)*

Honorable President George W. Bush

Mr. Kofi Annan *(Former UN Secretary General)*

(The Late Mr. John D. Rockefeller – An exception for "LATE" contributors to Global Health)

Other Healthcare related Organizations worth Commending for their tireless effort to seek the wellbeing of our global Citizenry and the USA in Particular:

NIH – National Institute of Health (USA)

CDC – Center for Disease Control (USA)

FDA – Food and Drug Administration (USA)

WHO – The World Health Organization (UN)

The Bill & Melinda Gates Foundation
(Philanthropic Organization)

The Clinton Foundation

(Philanthropic Organization)

The Kofi Annan Foundation

(Philanthropic Organization)

The Rockefeller Foundation

(Philanthropic Organization)

- The myriad of Global Contemporaries, in Collaborative Engagements relating to our general global health and well being. Which includes climate related health issues – Environmental Health, yet not forgetting all health workers nationally and globally and their patients.

All Academic Institutions doing the Same Globally, and especially my Alma Matters from elementary school, and Current Affiliate Institution, Faculty and Support Staff:

> Rutgers University – NJ
>
> New Jersey Institute of Technology – NJ
>
> The University of Ghana – Ghana
>
> Opoku Ware Secondary School – Ghana
>
> The State Experimental Primary School – Ghana

And Finally my Parents, Children, Teachers, and Pastors and well as Mentors and Friends. And also all business and institutions I have had the privilege and opportunity to both work for, and learnt from. I say all this in deep appreciation because I am a microcosm of all of these and more.

THE SYSTEMIC INTEGRATIVE THINKING APPROACHT TO PROBLEM SOLVINIG:

A Possible Paradigm [It's Application in Healthcare] and Obesity Prevention & Management.

(Health Informatics)

By

Kwasi Yeboah-Afihene

MAIN GOALS:

"Potential Creative Systemic Collaboration and Harmonized, safe, effective and cost contained solutions"

Preface

After watching an HBO program which was recorded in 2003 on the internet, about poor kids in America, with the title; "A boy's Life", I was quite saddened, yet encourage by the work I have chosen to do, which is starting with this book, at least to contribute a bit if any, to finding the way to debacle the OBESITY Myths and Mysteries. Or at least lead the way to those yet to be untied. It was about a family in Eudora, Mississippi.

The main character, or at least the focus of the story, was on a little boy, called Robert, and his family. An adorable little boy, caught in the middle of two different lives. As comfortable as we all deem home to be, for a normal little kid, Robert rather found school, a haven.

Not that there was anything so willfully designed to perpetuate that notion, he was simply a victim of some of the unfortunate, circumstance of life which he had little to do with, or little to even help himself otherwise.

Robert was a victim of teenage pregnancy. He was living in a house with his brother, mother and grandma. Though the family was seemingly supportive, at least to the best of their ability, which I believed from watching the video, was real in all their honest sincerity, at least his Grandma, who was supporting Robert, his brother and Mom.

Though the grandma was trying her very best as I initially mentioned, he had very little means, which afforded her also little freedom to do all that was needed, and necessary to make them all live the way little kids are suppose to, or perceived to be living normally by the general consensus of society.

Robert was perceived to be a troubled kid, though was in my opinion a very adorable kid, yet just a victim. In the home environment, which was poverty stricken, his behavior was influenced by the typical chronic stressors, which not only forces some unusual characteristics with some undesirable consequences, by even loved ones to the innocent they try so hard to protect and love.

The environmental nuances of Robert's home, through no one's willful design, impacted Robert so adversely that he had to go through a lot of unwarranted medical processes with ramifications that he really did not need.

At some point along the way, the people close to him as well as his social workers, realize that Robert was a very normal Kid. After close assessments of Roberts home environment, as it compared to his school environment, they found out that the problem was his home environment, because he was just fine elsewhere.

The reason why I am using this story is simply an example of some of the social effects or negative ripples that can emanate from childhood OBESITY. Though it can destroy an immediate victim, it can also affect very adversely the entire family.

Robert's mother was a teenage girl called Robbina. I do not know exactly the culprit of her behavioral issues, but I will not be surprised if it resulted from the most apparent effects of psychosocial impact of OBESITY. This can have a very devastating effect on even adults. Matured adult who may be more-savvy in dealing with the nuances of life, sometimes even get caught up with some of these negative psychosocial OBESITY related problems.

Knowing how brutal the High School or even elementary school environments can be for kids in general. For an OBESE kid in such an environment, it could be much more challenging. I am not condoning Robbina's seemingly anti-social behavior, nor do I blame it on anyone. However, I would be fairer to say both OBESITY and the lack of empathy of the school kids, who unknowingly create such an adversarial environment in the school, may have something to do with her lack of self-esteem, and other psychological problems which lead to such a behavior.

Also accelerated puberty which is sometimes characterized by obesity to children not yet matured for a normal age for puberty as we knew, could have also been a reason why, premature sexual indulgence which precipitated the birth of Robert came about.

Though, it will be easy to blame Robbina, for being very careless and a bad kid. If we will be honest with ourselves, when the wrong hormones kick in at the wrong time, even matured adults make similar mistake. For kids who have not matured enough, to even know and understand the causes and long term consequential effect of these stuff, and to add to that, with not much will power developed, or the awareness to abide even by the shadow of the Almighty, the punishment may be warranted but, deserves a lot of empathy.

Listening to Robbina and her mother, in some of their usual arguments, I could sense she was quite ambitious, though got side tracked early in life. The added burden, Robbina's behavior brought to the family was so tremendous than her mother Anna; a single mother could deal with single handedly with such little resources.

Robert then, was a victim of many things as I said earlier which were or not his fault. They said he has multiple personality, ADHD, and a slew of others. With the help of the social worker from the Department of Human Services at Mississippi, in collaboration with the school system, they realize that Robert was just a normal little kid, caught in between the demise of "Poverty, Obesity, Chronic Stress, Teenage Pregnancy, Divorce (Single Mother Grandma), and so on.

Eventually Anna could not hold on to the stress so much. Though not willingly, the body started giving up. She got terribly sick, with little hope for survival. The great end of the story is that, when her mother could no more hold on unfortunately, Robbina stepped up, and live up to her responsibility, and took care of the family including her own sick mother, though still young, yet a little bit more matured. The thought that came to mind was that, at least, if she had had the kids at that time, may be it would not have been that bad. She may have been wise enough to find a good responsible partner, or even worked as a single mother to help the kids better. These are some of the trends we should be watching also, as to the potential demise of obesity to our society and mankind in general, though there are a lot more equally deadly demises.

At that time, she was a bit matured enough to carry on. As good as the end of this story seems, not all of them end this way. Obesity indeed can destroy a generation, not only through physical ailments but also through many distortions in the psychosocial, socioeconomic, socio-cultural and geo-political domains in any country.

We often measure its impact primarily on cost of treatment and prevention, which is great. Yet the real issues, which are very long lasting and devastating to society as a whole, are hard to quantify with money. We therefore have to strike the right balance to our socio-economic domains as they relates to our pursuit of happiness and wellbeing.

That according to Adam Smith, who I will deem as the "Father of Economics" are the ultimate goals of these pursuits. Had it not been the love of the social worker from the "Department Of Human Services" and the School System, especially the dedication of a devoted Principal, we could all imagine, what the lives of Robert, brother and their mother, Robbina would have ended.

This story touched the innermost part of my heart. It ended this way though, not because the family was Caucasian or Indian, or Chinese or Black. This profile transcends that. It is a problem for all humanity. We are all in it together and have to work together to solve it, for the benefit of all. For that reason, I am not going to mention the ethnicity of the cast.

For all teenagers who get caught up in this or other similar situation, and for all parents and support families dealing with a similar situation. I would say do not lose heart. Keep loving, supporting and doing your very best for the victims and all the family members adversely affected. "To air is human", yet to some of these teenagers, they do not even have the maturity to soundly analyze either their environments or situations. They often just follow blindly in a dark alley. The issue only becomes apparent at the end of the tunnel, which is often too late, yet not so late, as Robbina's turned out to be. I believe there is hope.

Let us show empathy, and educate them well and early enough. Let us arm them, with the right information and understanding of these hidden risks. I believe it may not solve all the problems teenagers have, but will save a ton of them. Especially those which low self-esteem and peer pressure often triggers, which if not all, will cover the majority of their issues.

Acknowledgements

I will thank God, for his grace, love and protection. I also thank him for being the light of knowledge. My gratitude also goes to my Faculty advisers, Dr. Dinish Mital, and Dr. Shankar Srinivasan and Dr. Syed Haque, and also to my dear friend, Joyce Berko, and especially her husband, my "Fellow Katakyie", and senior in high school, Dr. Kofi Berko, who gave me the first thumps up with this idea.

I will also say thanks to Dr. Edward Achiampong, another" Fellow Katakyie" and senior, for the second thumps up. Then to another, Dr. Ernest Kwateng

Amankwa, my "Fellow Katakyie" but this time my own class mate in high school, for his usual help and encouragement. Then again another expression of gratitude to Dr. Kwadwo Ofori Ntim, Dr. Alex Quachie and Dr. Kofi Appiah, though of a rival high school, who claims to be the only Collage in town, I will also say thanks for all you do.

To a Fellow AISECER, Mr. Kofi Gyampo, "Fellow Katakyie" and a dormitory mate, Mr. Francis Afram-Gyening, Mr. Maxual Adjei a brother from Legon as well as Mr. Michel Kwateng, Mr. Prince Kena all legon mates and friends, Mr & Mrs. Kofi Anokye and Dr. Esi Abam, and lastly Mr.

Prince F. Kessie Esq. and Mr. William Blagogee Esq. I will say thanks also, for all you do.

Another thanks goes to all the supporting cast of my school and department. Especially the Library staff, which was like a second home to me, computing support staff and the entire faculty, and other administrative support staff of my department: The Health Informatics Department – Rutgers University – School of Health Related Services.

I will say thanks also to my cousin in Maryland whose house I stopped first before I left for the train station to head to DC to meet Dr. Kofi Berko. He said WOW, after I explained it first to him on my return from DC, though I knew he did not get it. I still say thanks Mr. Kwame Fosu. Kwame, my initial comment though was a JOKE, I know you got it!

To my family and friends who have been supportive in diverse ways, I will say thank you too. If I choose to mention the remaining names, I believe it could fill the book and have no space for the planned content. I also know you will understand. I would repeat though, thank to you all. Lastly to my Children, and former wife, who is helping them at home, I will also say thank you and God Bless you all.

Table of Contents

Introduction 34

Section I 73

Obesity 101 74

Obesity 201 103

The Pathogenesis of Metabolic Syndrome .. 162

Obesity Cost Outcomes 304

The Pathogenesis of Metabolic Syndrome in Children 360

Section II 384

The Systemic Integrative Thinking Approach to Problem
Solving……………………………………………………385

Introduction

Usually book dedications are not that long. Some of you may say that mine for this book was an over kill, yet after this peace, you may realize that it is really not after all, since it will all make sense in the end. To me, being a health worker is like home coming, and again I will tell you why latter.

I will start this way, though it may not be of interest to some of you of different inclinations toward religion and faith. What I am going to say has nothing to do with what I believe, though I do. I say so because the story fits in well with the example I am going to use. Its relevance is just contextually synergistic, though it is from the Bible.

They say or at least William Shakespeare says, "....to yourself be true." Sometimes, I wonder which self? Since we are a microcosm of many cultures, experiences, believes and others which replicate themselves in the "self" depending on circumstances and things we are sometimes confronted with. I say so not to talk about any diagnosis of multiple personalities and the likes. Pragmatism sometime calls for flexibility, practical flexibility, grounded in sound ethical and legal precepts are what work. Pardon me if my religious "self" peeks through here and there. That is not to annoy anyone. Though not making claims of being profound, it is just part of the mix of ingredients that constitutes my "self" which everyone says we should be true to.

I respect everyone's opinion and decisions regarding such issues, and I hope the nuances of mine will also be respected. The Bible says, teach a child what he should do, and even when he wonders away from it, he will always find his way back. This though is not quoted verbatim from any of its many translations; it is a re-phrase in my own words. The relevance of this though still remote, will become apparent in the next statement, I am going to make.

To me, being a health worker I believe is home coming, as I have said earlier. This is also going to clarify why I started the list of my Alma Matter from elementary school. At my elementary school, I was a student leader at one point. My area of leadership was in health and sanitation. I was responsible for making sure that the school's grounds sectioned for our group was clean before school starts in the morning. The groups were color coded and each color (Red, Yellow,

Green etc...) were responsible for making sure their respective grounds were free of litter. Every Friday, the best groups were hierarchically announces and honored. I cannot claim we won all the trophies, yet our group could safely pride ourselves of a lot of them.

That was where I started my health and sanitation work. Lots of time has passed, and I have really forgotten the color of the group that I was responsible for. My best guess though is either Red or Blue.

In High School, I was also very active in student government. I sent my nomination to the selection panel to include me as a candidate for Senior Prefect. This is like the president of the student council. After the panel of House Masters and the electoral committee, met and deliberated, they reshuffled the nominations.

My physics teacher, who was a house master, of St. Matthew's house, one of the student dormitories in our school, and our senior house master, the former house master for St. Mark's house, who is now diseased, came to me before the final nominations were announced. They told me that, Kwasi the panel think you could handle the health area better. I was a bit disappointed and said if that is the case, I may drop my nomination.

Very disappointed, the senior house master left. Mr. Owusu Mensah, who was the said physics teacher, pulled me on the side and spoke with me at length. Though it seems that I was a bit hard headed, I really wasn't. I am very principled when it comes to certain things, and I often stick to my guts if I believe I am doing the right thing, especially if I truly believe.

He finally told me, that he knew it is a very tough job, and they believe, I could handle it better amongst the submitted candidates. For his believe in me, I bent and took the honor. I did so, also because he indicated that it is an area help is well needed.

The Election Day came and went, and the long story short, I won the election with a decisive margin. I did not make much noise and did not even have a slogan like many of the other candidates who even had songs. How I did it, many of my rivals copied, including those contesting for the other positions. It was a very simple but effective strategy, which did not cost much. I would also say though, it was also by grace that it came to me. The second person was not even close. I really campaigned very hard to make sure I get the opportunity to serve in an area where help was most needed, by my superiors who believed in me.

The health prefect was in charge of the school's clinic and a liaison for students, making sure their interest was well served. It was quite a big student population and also a boarding Catholic School. Our team of three health prefect of which I was the senior, (Oscar Papa Ntim, and Richid Boamah) had the responsibility of making sure all the classrooms including the teachers' lounges and offices were clean including the grounds. We collaborate very effectively and worked hard every day, to make sure the school's grounds were spanking clean every morning, before school start. That often meant waking up earlier than the typical wake up time of most students to make sure what is needed done gets done and on time. We also had to make sure the school clinic was operating to the best interest of the general student population.

By the way, my position only rivaled with the senior prefect position, since we were the only ones amongst the student leadership group that had two partners to work with.

This work was schedule and divided amongst a lot of the junior students from grade three and down. We were therefore in charge of more than half of the student population, making sure everyone does what they were suppose to do before school starts.

Sometimes we met most of our expected outcomes, and sometimes, we miss by a few. For the students who do not do their respective assigned work, we find the best way to punish them so they become more responsible next time. This job was during my last two years of high school when I was preparing for my advanced level GCE, to go to college. In college I wanted to go to either the pharmacy school or the medical school. Long story short, I did not get either, and I will not blame it on my busy schedule with the junior students, I just guess it was not meant to be, at least at that time.

Missing the opportunity to become a health worker, I was a bit disillusioned, about college. As a result it was not that fun to me. Though my Dad wanted me to go to engineering school, I was not very interest in his proposition, because I did not think that was my calling. He wanted me to, because he had some connections in the mining industry in Ghana which he thought could get me in, after school and then go to graduate school to study business administration.

I realized after all that was the best instinctive choice, otherwise I may have been bunging heads with my own brother, Kwame Ado-Kuffour who is now head the mining company my Dad had in mind. Kwame, if you get a copy of this book, I hope you get a good laugh. May be, one good turn deserves another. I tried chemistry, yet my heart was not in the pure sciences, though I loved chemistry in high school. There I did more than the typical number of courses, combining the sciences and liberal arts. After leaving the University of Science and Technology in Kumasi, I settled for Economics and Computer Science as a Liberal arts dual combination, though I was also accepted in the Book Industry Program at the UST (The University of Science and Technology).

Whether books and healthcare which I missed in a greater part of my career life was a destiny, which showed up a bit early as a prophetic sign for what has heightened my passion now, I do not know, though it may have been.

In the University of Ghana, where I studied Economics and Computer Science, I was also very active in another student organization. Though not political as the other student leadership affiliations, it was rather business focus. Whiles in college, I had the opportunity to work with my Dad many times who was a business man. In fact he thought me a lot consciously and unconsciously. I say unconsciously, because many of the times he did not even know I was learning anything from him.

I learnt more from observing what he did and how he did it, even more than what he formerly instructed me to do.

Most of what I picked from his instruction was tough words of wisdom. I say tough because I did not understand then, until I grew up. That is when I learnt the practicality of what he was getting at. He often said, live for a purpose, whatever that is, business is just to serve the needs of people, if that is what you want to do, if you serve their needs well enough, you will be ok.

The organization I was affiliated with was AIESEC. With the help of some insider friends in the organization (Kwame Addo-Kuffour and Andrew Osei Akoto), I managed to navigate well to become one of the national leaders of the organization.

My area of leadership was Projects. I was the Vice President for AIESEC Ghana in charge of Projects. Most of these projects were international seminars which we organized and invited fellow "AIESECERS" all over the world.

Though I say was a bit disillusioned with college, because of not getting the opportunity to become a doctor or a pharmacist, AIESEC filled in the void. I was very active fund raising, than studying. It may sound funny, but it was true. I was saved though by a few friends who had a very good command on the English Language, coupled with an excellent penmanship.

Barbara Coleman was one of them. Barbara was a very pretty girl and also very personable. Though she had a boy friend then, there were other secret admirers, one of whom was a colleague, Awuah Darko. Though Sweve as he was called then, was not ranking that high in queue, though he was a bit aggressive forcing his way to get ahead in queue.

I did not even attempt to nurture my intent to be in line, because I thought it as a waste of time. I therefore just maintained my lead position in the study mate queue, because that was serving me well, especially in catching up on school work after a busy AIESEC related fundraising errands or travel.

I know, both Barbara and Sweve will laugh at the last paragraph, when they happen to see this, though a nice joke to reminisce the good old days back in Legon. I do not feel guilty now, because I did not sin. I was a bit close though, by just pondering joining the secret admirers queue momentarily. This makes me laugh, and I think it would make most of you do the same.

Fast forwarding, I got into technology here in the USA, after graduate school at NJIT. I am proud of the school, because I think they prepared me well, and were also helpful, especially the career development department, in helping me land some internships, and finally my AT&T job through their famous job fair, which bring a lot of big conglomerates as well as medium to small businesses on campus.

At the end of my career with AT&T, I decided to get into business for myself. Amongst other endeavors, I settle with Insurance and banking as an insurance agent for one of the very iconic USA insurance companies.

(Allstate Insurance Co.)

After incubating my business and getting it off to an accelerated growth rate, I met an uncertainty that reversed the successes I worked so hard to build. The period I am talking about is most familiar to many. The economic tsunami that swept our land, taking on giant like Bears Stern and many in the banking and Insurance industry, which force them to tighten up, made business quite challenging, and almost impossible. With cash flow tightening up also as a result, my current ratio was just not workable, at least for my operations.

With the end site of the storm too far off, and its apparent difficult uncertainty still looming, I had to make a very hard business decision to execute an exit plan to at least salvage whatever I could, before the whole pot tumbles over. In the process, I quickly learnt that, what business schools, have to spend more time on is the business exit plans, and how to execute. Incubating business is fun, but losing your baby and having no one's sympathy but you alone and also be the only one at the funeral, if you are lucky to have a priest with you, is not that fun.

In spite of the lose, I did not give up. I wanted to restructure the business in a different format. After an extreme hard work with not much capital, or facilities for leverage, I decided to be more creative and form another organization that I thought could help support the Insurance brokerage I was incubating, apparently with nothing much.

I managed to go far with both businesses little by little. In the process, the auxiliary business became my passion and that was the initial home coming into the healthcare industry. It was a healthcare business concept for the aged.

The concept was to create an environment, to help families better manage their elderly parents who may not be in close proximity due to economic dispersion and work obligations that sometime take us out of our home state. The idea was to create a safe and easily manageable synergistic collaboration amongst, medical as well as custodial caregivers, the family members and the elderly. Also with the respective agencies and institutions who provide resources and personnel helping and facilitating the process of care giving for the elderly, through a web portal and physical support staff. I was going to model it in NJ, with the hope of extending it beyond after perfecting the business model.

I also had a part that was meant to enhance social interactions amongst family members, to improve their distance relationships, at least for Grandmas, and Grandpas, to have some fun with their grand children and other family members' afar, on the internet.

After the process of concept formulation and development was getting far along the way, I became again even more anemic. I hope most business folks understand the relation of blood and money as it relate to life of humans and that of businesses. After pushing it to my wits end, I finally had to give up. This healthcare business was hosted at the NJIT- CDC. Which is a great small business incubation center in our area, and definitely the best of its kind in NJ, if not the north east.

When I threw in the towel in business, brook and busted, with all kinds of financial woes, I still did not give up. I decided to go back to school and improve my academic and business competencies in Healthcare. Given my background, I thought health informatics was a good marriage.

After wondering and meandering for a while, my faculty advisers guided me to a niche that has consumed my passion. I started with cancer, but seeing the magnitude of the problem related to OBESITY, and the requisite cost to society and mankind in general, my passion kind of heightened along that path. After a while I was flip flopping as usual with PhD programs, about where to land the boat. I was fluctuating between Public Health, Management, Payer and Cost related issues or clinical issues.

After combing the literature a bit, I realize that most problems were not necessary clinical, especially what I can draw from my background and experiences to make a difference in the field. I know I was very analytical in addition to other soft and hard requisite skills, but where to land was quite tough to discern, though OBESITY and other co-mortifies and related problems were certain.

Again, my advisers were very helpful, but thought I was hard headed sometimes. I truly was not any of those. I was thinking that if I am going to spend the time, it got to be well spent. I was very determined to make a significant difference as I often told our department chair, even as early as my admission interview for the program.

Not necessarily too big of a thing, but something that can be useful and meaningful to many. I read quite a bit about the subject and related problems yet could not come to any real conclusions about the landing field, which will heighten the usefulness of my little contribution.

I spoke to every PhD friend I have, including some of my friends and family members who were medical practitioners. I still could not pin down on anything. One day I decided to go to Maryland to talk to a friend, a senior in high school and the husband of a good friend. He was at work then, in DC. I visited a cousin in Maryland and managed to leave my car at his residence, and find a public transportation to my friend's office, which is a US government agency in down town DC.

In fact I have forgotten which agency it was, but on my way to DC, I was still thinking about my new baby OBESITY. It was in the train that the idea of the Systemic Integrative thinking approach to problem solving was born, at least in my head. I took my exercise book, and a pen in the train, and started pouring the ideas down as it came to me.

In a rainy day in DC, a little soaked yet my books intact because of my little hand bag, I finally saw my friend, Dr. Kofi Berko. I showed Kofi, what I had just come up with in the train. He looked at it, and was a bit enthused by it. His affirmation of the idea gave me some confidence that it may be useful. Upon my return to NJ, I showed to another friend to see what he has to say. His name is Dr. Edward Acheampong, who works as a research scientist at Rutgers, on several AIDS related issues.

He jumped on the idea and said it was supper. If you need help, I can help you. I then scheduled an appointment with my advisers, regarding my new idea. It was a fun meeting. They though liked it but questioned its scope and practical implementation within the time period I was planning to graduate, and also its funding.

I was a bit saddened, because I really did not want to let go. Fast forwarding to now, I have at least found a way of developing it further, and especially apply it in solving or helping get us along the way on the right tangent, regarding our quest for solution with the OBESITY epidemic. Hence this series of books as the first step to further develops the concept by expanding it, free flow.

I chose to do it this way in order to get the input of many, and also give people the opportunity to experience it in simple language and have the opportunity to help in its development. As long as it may take, every one's input will be paramount in perfecting it, at least at whatever state or destination I bring it, by his grace. I believe, solutions from pure academic setting set good boundaries, but it takes every stakeholder, including patients or prospective patients which include all of us, to bring out its most essential pragmatic gems.

That is one of the reasons for publishing this work this way, at the onset of the concept formulation. That will also give me the chance to think through more thoroughly and also learn along the way, without much restriction imposed by academic boundaries, though the scrutiny and discipline is the most critical piece that will get it thoroughly examined, and scientifically developed for any useful engagements regarding the concept.

I will after this project, tighten it with literature and present it in an academic journal to start the debate there also, with the help of my faculty advisers. The first thing I did with this project was to create electronically my scribbles in multiple notebooks. After that was done, I shared it with a few important people in the healthcare debate. Just so they get an early start with the idea, including my mentors and advisers.

After all, they are the ones that can really make a real difference with it. It may not be a totally new idea, I do not know, but I came up with it, drawing from a life time of experiences and studies. I believe also that it all came together by HIS grace. By "HIS", I mean God. I hope I do not have to caution again, for this is just my belief.

As I have already said, it is just my belief, which is an integral piece of my "SELF", which is better always to be true to. I however want this work to be judged by the soundness of its rational, logical and practical tenets with good scientific precept. Since it has to be categorized under science, either social or others, my belief does not conflict with science. I am also a scientist, as it related to my academic work.

I will then integrate the final concept into my research proposal for further studies. I have written a couple of books, ["ADVACED ANALITICS: A New Healthcare Management Informatics

Apparatus: – "An Overview" (English Version)", "Little Blue Inspirational Series Vols: 1 – 6", "Little Blue Preventive Medicine Series: Cancer", The Demise of Aging, "Identity Crises" and more....] which as I said initially, was probably where the initial book industry admission at UST, which I "passed", signified. I hope you enjoy the reading and most importantly, share your thought and ideas with me.

It will be in two sections. One describing OBESITY and health related issues, and the other; summarizing "Creative Systemic Integrative Thinking Approach to Problem Solving, as it relates to healthcare in general and OBESITY specifically. This section is going to be as brief as I can, but with enough content to bring out its meaning and intended goals. The fully developed concept will be presented to the best of my ability God willing, and all the help I can get in the second version of this series. At least, the best I can do now is describing it well enough for you to understand its description.

I however need a lot of input to ascertain the practical nuances of the models I have so far. For that reason, let us just hold our breath, and time to work it through together. I strongly believe, it will take many minds to get it where it could be pragmatically useful. I also hope as I believe you all do, that is the end we are all wishing, or hoping to reach. Hopefully the obesity epidemic will be on its way to extinction. This though will only be possible, if we all put our heads and ideas together to drive it out, with creative systemic collaborative engagements.

SECTION I

OBESITY 101

I will start this section with a quote from Wikipedia. I like definitions from Wiki, because they are usually very simple. Their usual user friendliness enhances its usefulness, and functional stands, because it is usually easily understood by many readers from all walks of life. Though not advertising for Wiki, it is true, at least for me and many others that I have referred to.

Most people though question the authenticity of some of their content sometime, yet I would say that, with my experience with them, they are just fine most of the time, is not all. It mostly gives you the general knowledge and overview needed most of the time. Sometimes, for real academic work they may or may not be that useful, since the real sources of their work lack the critical scrutiny sometimes needed for academic research. It may however be ok for definitions and stuff though, as in this case.

Regarding obesity, I do understand some of the underlining factors. I would therefore say, with this writing and the breath of its intended audience, Wiki is quite on target. I however, do not by this statement claim any responsibility for any liabilities that may result from the usage of this or any information from Wiki. For any issue which required serious commitment of any kind, or that can adversely affect health. Or can inflict any damage or pain, for such endeavors that may pose even the slightest indication of such risks, please for your own protection; seek the appropriate professional advice and counsel. If this advice is ignored, any liability or negligence, which results in the usage of such information or in fact any in this book, may be on you. Again, Please seek the appropriate professional help for any health or anything that can create loses or pain to you or anyone.

I quote:

"Obesity is a medical condition in which excess body fat has accumulated to the extent that it may have a negative effect on health, leading to reduced life expectancy and/or increased health problems. People are considered obese when their body mass index (BMI), a measurement obtained by dividing a person's weight by the square of the person's height, exceeds 30 kg/m2.

Obesity increases the likelihood of various diseases, particularly heart disease, type 2 diabetes, obstructive sleep apnea, certain types of cancer, and osteoarthritis. Obesity is most commonly caused by a combination of excessive food energy intake, lack of physical activity, and genetic susceptibility, although a few cases are caused primarily by genes, endocrine disorders, medications or psychiatric illness. Evidence to support the view that some obese people eat little yet gain weight due to a slow metabolism is limited. On average obese people have greater energy expenditure than their thin counterparts due to the energy required to maintain an increased body mass.

Dieting and physical exercise are the mainstays of treatment for obesity. Diet quality can be improved by reducing the consumption of energy-dense foods such as those high in fat and sugars, and by increasing the intake of dietary fiber. Anti-obesity drugs may be taken to reduce appetite or decrease fat absorption when used together with a suitable diet. If diet, exercise and medication are not effective, a gastric balloon may assist with weight loss, or surgery may be performed to reduce stomach volume and/or bowel length, leading to feeling full earlier and a reduced ability to absorb nutrients from food.

Obesity is a leading preventable cause of death worldwide, with increasing rates in adults and children. Authorities view it as one of the most serious public health problems of the 21st century. Obesity is stigmatized in much of the modern world particularly in the Western world, though it was widely seen as a symbol of wealth and fertility at other times in history, and still is in some parts of the world. In 2013, the American Medical Association classified obesity as a disease." [Wikipedia]

Obesity is both a clinical and public health issue. For an individual, it poses clinical issues, and for a bigger population, either a country or our global landscape as a whole, a public health issue. Clinician, and other caregivers, as well as manufacturers and practitioners in related trades, and industries all help to work hard to meet the needs of patients with such health issues. The consequences of Obesity though, transcend the individual victims. Its impact can affect a whole nation and even, the global community at large. Here is a summary of some thoughts and related issues:

- Obesity, its related co-morbidities, and the cost outcomes have huge negative monetary, social as well as psychological effects which are currently ballooning in its adverse consequential outcomes.
- If not controlled, could send the global healthcare systems and associated economies, and societies into a pandemonium.
- The pain and suffering to humanity which could likely result from a

health epidemic of such magnitude, is very much avoidable.

- My philosophical or value tangent in this debate, which I believe is the most cost effective and efficient way to address the issue, is via prevention. This thought, sterns most eminently, from wellness living (Making good Lifestyle choices, regarding almost every aspect of your health, by totally participating in the total management of one's health, which may also require the collection and understanding of all their vital statistics, relating to their current health conditions or potential known, health predispositions) and thinking, knowing the risk factors.

- It is commonly believed that the addictive nature of the factors that affect the human energy controls, which when create a surplus, store excess energies as fats and extra body tissues, often as in Obesity.
- This has some merit, but evidently not a sustainable and dominant cofactor in the mix of many.
- The different paradigms, and schools of thought on how obesity is formed, and how best it can be controlled, kind of create a cognitive dissidence, given its mainly unsustainable and unpredictable outcomes.
- Obesity, creates a pathway for many other diseases, some of

which are fatal and others, slow killers with high maintenance and equally fatal. The only differences being a longer lease hold on poor quality of life. In order words, it is a bio-marker for a lot of other diseases that are triggered by the same human internal mechanisms that affect our fat accumulation and body weight, when they get out of hand.

- The question then is: what can be discovered in the current obesity healthcare data and literature, which can help researcher to find safe, efficable and economically sound pharmacological or non pharmacological remedies, given a good understanding of the risk factors. Such remedies could help break or restrain the pathway to obesity. This I believe will in turn restrain the pathways to many of its, related co-morbidities, improving ultimately the quality of life of patience, and healthcare cost outcomes in general.

- From the work done so far, I am more inclined to believe that, amongst the various cofactors in the competing mix of schools of thoughts, a proper balanced diet with less carbohydrates, especially sugar and a good understanding of our human physiology, especially pertaining to the follow systems and bodies of knowledge, will go a long way in providing the insightful prerogatives needed to debacle the puzzle:

- The digestive system
- The endocrine system and how it affects our metabolism, especially pertaining to the accumulation of fat in our fat cell. (Identifying the dominant related subsystems)
- The main food groups and major ingredients of digestive outcomes that constitute the main triggers which adversely affect the processing and storage of fat.

- Genetic predisposition and the role it plays in fat accumulation and processing.
- The nervous system and how it regulates to the addictive behaviors of humans, even when we are aware of serious adverse side effect.
- Nutrition Science
- Coronary Art and Science
- Lifestyle & related Activities
- Agriculture practices
- Food Processing industry
- Pharmaceutical Industry
- Exercise and recreational Sports Industry

- Healthcare Industry in general
- Restaurant and Other related food Industry
- Food Manufacturers
- Environmental Health Sciences
- Sociology/Anthropology
- Economics/Finance
- Education
- Etc.

A very critical analysis of related data and literature can reveal a wealth of knowledge that can have a great impact on the entire global healthcare ecosystem. I believe there are some physiological, socio-economic, geo-political and other anthropological factors that researchers are missing. These internal and external factors looked at holistically; I believe will merge Science, Technology and the Humanities at the right equilibrium to produce sustained results or outcomes.

I also believe that Informatics is an integrative science which requires creative systemic integrative thinking. It primarily merges the medical sciences and technology to produce the best models and decision support systems and procedures that ultimately improves clinical and administrative outcomes. It is in this light that I believe a creative systemic integrative and collaborative view of the health informatics domain, obesity and healthcare in general should be paramount in our quest for sustainable healthcare solutions. It will help us come with the best models, and ultimately, sustainable and sound outcomes especially as expected.

Some related tools may have to be innovated though some are here already. These technological advancements can be a technology accelerator to spear head the momentum into a different more favorable direction. Some of these will emanate from: Related Scientific and Academic literature, Mathematical & Statistical Competencies, and related Data. Also related IT and advanced analytics tools yet to be identified or even well known.

Socio-Cultural Trends Relating to OBESITY.

The issue with the accumulation of fat, in our adipose tissues, which when, become excessive "mutates" our usual physic into a little bigger form, through the progressive gaining of weight if not properly controlled is the health phenomena called obesity. The process of becoming obese twists a bit, the ratio used to mathematically depict our body mass, as it relates to our normal height which is typically pegged below 30 units, with any above that threshold considered obese: The BMI [body mass index], as our initially quoted article in Wiki described.

Obesity rates or simply the general size of our population, in relationship to our height, is getting a bit disproportional, within healthy limits, as acceptable by medical experts. That is, the normal related healthy weight and size proportions are getting a bit outside of our known healthy standards acceptable by the medical and healthcare ecosystem.

As a result, there are a lot of related health indications, with numerous monetary and other inherent economic negative ramifications, nationally and globally. This does not even measure the other related psychosocial/emotional and other outcomes that adversely affects our wellbeing, happiness and productivity in general.

The overall impact is insurmountably scary, when properly understood. It is like a Tsunami, heading our way, yet, worse than it, in terms of catastrophic impact on humanity in General.

The unfortunate situation as we have, or at least some of us have observed, is the socio-economic trends popping up here and there, to perpetuate it. The Obesity rates started it's ascend in the 80s. It has however, gathered momentum since, at a rate of acceleration which is quite stunning. What is most needed is a trend that rather force a descend.

If the climax is not here already, then it is very scary. Some of these trends though are as a result of the victims of

OBESITY forcing their social acceptance into the mainstream of society.

The societal resistance and sometimes the apparent mockery of them, forces on them a myriad of psychosocial adverse consequences. Some of these may be related to self-esteem and other emotional indications. Their resistance to accepting these forced psychosocial adverse impacts inflicted on them by society, they foster their own acceptance or isolated coalition, socializing within, and creating an economic force which naturally become an attraction for economic gain buy businesses created to meet such needs.

I do not blame it on the business men nor the obese population, but rather, I believe that society should be a little more sensitive to the demise of others, especially the victims of OBESITY.

If not, the society as a whole and even posterity will suffer a great deal. This is true because women, being the bearers of life, unfortunately or fortunately, set the pace of the future health of posterity. Though not single handedly, regarding obesity and related issue, they have the most impact. For instance from, child birth rates to childhood obesity, they practically dictates the outcomes for generations to come.

A baby's birth rate primarily is related to their mother's weight during and even before pregnancy. This could then be carried by the baby, through his life path, if not intervened early enough. Besides, they control also to a large extent home economics, nutrition and dietary need of most families. They even control the activity levels of children, in terms of even partying and sports activities for most children. As a result of that, I think we should socially be responsible at least for women's health issues directly or indirectly through public health initiatives. It can be a very good starting point to start reversing the trend. Their issue carries more potential ripples in society which transcends them, and even the current generation.

The following are a few of the related socio-economic and other related trends:

➢ Obese Population Self Acceptance Movements

➤ Modeling and Fashion Statements Marketing that Fat is beautiful. It is true that all things are beautiful in their own rights, beauty is not the issue. It is about health, wellbeing and happiness. What would you rather choose; A beautiful or handsome person, who spends all his resources on medicine or hospital bills, as oppose to the same, yet with a little preventive and health management adjustments can improve health, and rather enjoy their resources on things that are more fun, or even have more impact on them, family or even the future generation. I will leave that decision for each individual.

- Increase in self destructive struggle to get accepted through the disregard of body weight and healthy dietary guidelines.
- Adult sports/prostitutions with the obese.
- Social clubs and support groups for the obese.
- 19 Million People with phobias relating to the fear of being thin.
- Ergonomic modifications for a ton of industries, including but not limited to:
    - Transportation
    - Air Travel Industry
    - Hospitals
    - Furniture Manufacturing
    - Home building and design

- Work related ergonomic modifications
- Occupational Health
- Workers Compensation issues
- Cost of group health insurance for businesses
- Business Productivity
- Cost of Labor and Goods in general
- Tardiness and Health and absenteeism related to general mobility and negative health outcome due to obesity related problems.

➢ Pampering ourselves with food as well as our children.

- Over indulgence in eating due to chronic stress and other related problems.
- Over indulgence due to past trauma.
- Adverse effect on children due to obesity related mobility issues.
- Food and excessive eating to celebrate almost every occasion.
- A new dating trend called Feederism – Where the fiancée just help the other partner to get bigger and bigger.
- Psychological Aberration
- Cheap unhealthy industrial Diet

I will end this section with a joke. But before, I will share my sentiment and concern with the current trends in obesity rates globally. After reading a summary of WHO report on obesity rate in continental Europe, I was really stunned with the statistical report.

Though I know the issue is quite extensive globally, my expectation on Europe was a bit favorable. I thought it was not as bad. This notion though came from a historical perception I had.

Now the joke:

"When foreign travel become quite common in Africa, most of the fortunate ones who got the chance to travel abroad, saw something great they came to share. They said, there are wonderful and great looking blonds in Europe. In fact most people changed their persecution of what an appropriate physic should be.

Dieting became a trend for many, though we always historically thought being a bit heavy is sexy. I am not being insensitive, but I just want us all to have a little brake and laugh or smile a little.

When I saw the new statistics, I was stunned. The oxymoron thought was that, I was a bit confused about what was really sexy. Or who is setting the trend now. Ie. Who is following who? Well, the only saving grace in all of this was that, I learnt that at least the Swiss and the French are still pushing the old fashion healthy trends. Though we beat them with the language and some other stuff, I think they got us on this one."

Folks, with all seriousness, we need also to find a better way to deal with this obesity epidemic situation.

OBESITY 201

Most of the discussion here in this section, was drawn mostly from a TV program, recoded from the University of California. However it was distributed in "Youtube". There may be other ideas drawn from different sources but primarily, the most salient points were from the show, though some of them I was familiar with from other sources.

The looming cloud of the Obesity epidemic, in pandemic proportions is quite clear at this point, so far as its menses to individuals and the entire society is concerned. As I said before, there are many schools of thoughts. From improper dietary and nutritional consumption and related issues, inactive live styles, to genetics and metabolic issues, it is somehow difficult to explain the obesity rate in babies that often leads also to childhood obesity.

As I said earlier, this can only be explained by the metabolic and other nutritional habits of the mother, which pass on to the baby even before a safe delivery. Just to reiterate, by the very important point made earlier, obesity in women should be very carefully looked at. They are at least the most influential, factor that can make the most difference in our quest to tilt the tide. Not that the other factors are not important. Though they all are, the overreaching negative consequential nuances and ripples their impact can cause, way exceeds any other co-factor.

Divorce, which has precipitated many cultures and related extra busy lifestyles for most custodial parents, sometime leaves them and the kids also to the mercy of some of these unhealthy trends. This more often than not, exacerbates the growth rate of the obesity epidemic. The attractiveness of such activities is due to convenience and cost, or sometimes just the only option available.

It is a well known fact that cabs or calories in general are bad. Most people through the advice of experts started counting cab, and reduced their caloric intake. This advice holds some truths. But inherent in the truth is also a lot of chuff. Why I say so is that, not all calories are bad for the body. The body also needs cabs as well. After an extensive look into the big word "Cabs" and "Calories", the worse culprit was sugar and stuff that turns into sugar during its digestive processes easily and quickly. With sugar highest in that hierarchy, polished grains comes next. The easier the food groups turn into sugar, the worse it is, as it relate to fueling the accumulation of fat in related body cells. The fat content of food though has a role to play, still does not rank as high and sugar and easily digestible cabs that turns into sugar ultimately relatively quickly.

I am not advocating that sugar is poisonous to the body. It is really not, however, we need to exercise a bit of caution and be sparingly moderate in its consumption. Most often the additional quantity that tips us over the edge is mostly discretionary. Such as most sugar sweetened sodas and snakes. The level of moderation is per individual; depending on their own metabolic and genetic predispositions of related body processes, needs and indications.

Medical indications that can be triggered buy your body's intolerance for excessive sugar consumption like diabetes and so on should be watched carefully. Mostly they can be contained by strict and appropriate nutritional habits, sometimes with the help of related experts in the diet and nutrition field. This though has to be accessed individually. If you have a family problem relating to metabolic syndrome, especially diabetes, it may serve you well to shy away from the excessive consumption of sugar in general or the discretionary source of sugar as I have already mentioned.

The following are examples of health indications that can result from metabolic syndrome:

- ➤ Type 2 Diabetes
- ➤ Hypertension

- Lipid Problem (eg. High cholesterol and related issues)
- Cardiac Diseases

These metabolic syndrome related indications, unfortunately, forms the biggest chunk of chronic or non infectious diseases, which unfortunately have the highest cost component in our healthcare budget, relating to their management and treatment globally. It is so because of how it deeply permeates our demographics across all socio-economic profiles, and also across age cohorts.

These are other obesity related co-morbidities that are also costly monetarily and others:

➢ Non Alcoholic Fatty Acids

➢ Liver complications

➢ Dementia

➢ Cancer

➢ Polyphonic Ovarian Syndrome

➢ Etc

The combination of all these Obesity related health problems, takes a big toll on the aggregate global health cost. It takes as much as 75% approximately. The unfortunate part though is that, it is still struggling hard to gain "MARKET SHARE". The fact though is that, the pie is not getting bigger resource wise. What then are we going to give up for their gain in "Market Share". We have to start thinking really seriously about it. The opportunity cost either way is huge.

I do not want to through a lot of obesity related number at you, because I have a lot of friends that are allergic to numbers, especially when you hint them that they were mathematically deduced. I therefore do not want to lose anyone. I will rather recommend that you may have more fun finding your own related numbers that may make sense to you. Start with your family, your friends, school mates, office mates, co-workers, church family, and so on. If you do not have an enticing number, that will excite your counting genius, whenever you go to Disney or Universal studio, or any amusement part to have fan, at your roller coaster breaks or lunch breaks, just take a short peak by the food court. I bet if you are a real numbers person, you may not go on any other ride.

If you have the passion I do have, or the empathy for those you are counting, you may suddenly end your vacation. You cannot ride on any roller coaster, with tears, especially if not that of joy. I hope though that as winding as I have been, with this point, you still understand what I mean. If this triggers laughter, please just stop it. This is really nothing to laugh at, at least till the next real joke.

To throw in another number which you may be familiar with earlier, it is from when I mentioned earlier regarding the onset of the obesity rate's accelerated ascend. That number if you remember is 80's. Coincidentally, 80% of obese people are unhealthy. Most of them have diseases such as described earlier. The United Nation recently alerted that, non communicable diseases, in order word, such obesity related chronic and other diseases, posses a much more danger than communicable (Infectious diseases) to the developing world. If you have an idea, of the crippling impact of communicable diseases on the developing world, I bet I can stop the plead here, regarding the apparent sense of urgency we need to attach to this issue globally.

I though the issue was much more serious here in the USA. Then they said Europe is also bleeding. Now they are saying again the developing world. I know a little bit of math, hence the reason why most of my friends are allergic to mathematically deduced numbers. I remember though, my "abc" from kindergarten, as well as my 1+1 =2 and my first phonics book, "SO-so", in elementary school. I do not even have to draw from any high school math skill and beyond. Even, with the little math I remember from elementary school, what they are talking about is primarily the whole world. "A little laughter brake".

I mentioned earlier that sugar, intake that exceeds your bodies needs, can be very dangerous. The reason being that, the two major components of sugar, being Glucose and Fructose, though needed by the body, could also harm it.

I know there are more social science student than those in the hard sciences. I will therefore be fair by making my explanation of the role sugar play very simple. I want to make it so, also because I want my own life also to be simple. Why because, Mr. William Gates save me by including spell check in MS Word. I did not do too well in elementary school with my spelling B. I also did not care too much about spelling in high school because I was using numbers more often than I had to spell. It caught up with me though, when I started my liberal arts education in the University of Ghana.

To be fair with each other, I think it will be better to keep it simple. Simple so you understand, and so I do not have to struggle with the spelling of some of these words that are even a mouth full pronouncing.

In short, excess fructose puts more pressure on the liver, and also triggers excess insulin. Glucose also works with it, but fructose is the worse culprit. Insulin is a hormone, whatever that is. I said that because I just wanted to be a bit funny. Again, to keep it simple, insulin plays a very vital role in the way the body works internally. It is like a quarter back, if you understand the American football.

It affects almost every aspect of the way the endocrine system works, especially in the case of obesity, how fat is metabolized and finally stored in the appropriate body cells. The body needs insulin to work very efficiently for all the related part to follow. Just as an ineffective or inefficient quarter back can really "screw up" a game, so is ill regulated Insulin.

Excessive consumption of sugar, overworks the liver in the process of metabolizing glucose and fructose, which needs insulin. Over producing it beyond safe limits, leads to improper regulated insulin production and function, which affects the way it plays its role as a quarter back. This as we all well know, or can assume if we know the role of a quarter backs, will definitely mess the game.

I do not want to confuse you with a lot of medical and scientific terminologies, yet I hope you very well understood the explanation giving with the football example. Essentially, all that I was saying was that, anything that adversely affects the healthy production and functioning of insulin can also do the same to your health to a large extent. If you really got it, then that was great. I used football because most of us understand that game, at least in the USA. I know lots of people elsewhere may prefer soccer, but it just do not fit well in this analogy, just to be fair. Even some of us that only relates to it during the super bowl get it to some extent. If well enough to let you get these complex phenomena that well, then I at least I did ok.

When the whole process gets a bit off course, as I have already described, then is when all these ugly head show up. I simply mean metabolic syndrome related indications as well as all or most of the other indications I presented earlier. Be very careful though with sugar, since as sweet as it is, it could also be very costly. I think this is more than you need to know, before I lose you, since it can actually get very complicated otherwise.

The last point to note before I finally stop this section is quite a scary thought. Over a long period of time, liver transplants have been due to damages caused by hepatitis. Unfortunately liver fat which ultimately causes it to stiffen has taken over. This also is a result of obesity and related cohort's adiposity, resulting from metabolic syndrome.

The next question is why our body size started getting bigger and bigger, all of a sudden after the 80's and beyond. The answer may not be that simple. There may be a major culprit, but whether it is the main cause or a response to phenomena engendered by something else, or simply a response to a need, is not quite certain. We often blame obesity on the Western Industrial diet, which turn out to be unhealthy, though responding to our cry for hunger.

What then caused the need or pain they served, or mutated its expected outcomes so of tangent? The little I know about business, they are formed to fill a void or serve a need. Everyone points at McDonalds and the likes, but we may first have to point may be to our "taste buds". Though they are a co-factor in the issue, the axiomatic cause, which engendered that need and the form of the solution, if still prevalent in our environment, should be seriously addressed. That may present some actionable insights to get us along the right direction, if we really need a better solution, or is just crying out loud.

Every business model that I know is not written in stone, especially in this hyper dynamic and overheated global economic environment like we have today. The Harvards, Oxfords, Yales, Rutgers, NJIT, Legon and the likes, teach their business students to be flexible, and tune their ear closely to their overall business environments and adjust accordingly. In fact I think they do, in obedience to the genius of these great "Alma Matters" and their first hand experience with the brutal fact of the realities on the ground.

My little "MINI" CEO title I had, for a brief period of time, gave me some empathy for business leaders. Though some are crocked, like any profession, I strongly believe most aren't. If you really understand what it takes to get business operations going in this overheated hyper dynamic economic environment moving at the speed of light, the next time you meet your CEO, I mean a real one, not my MINI example, you will just smile and say Hi, to boost his or her spirit. It is sometimes more than a Doggy Dog World out there. If he comes home safe, at least with a week's pay check, just say thanks, with all sincerity. I say this with lots of empathy for them, from my own personal experience when hell started braking loose in my business.

If I were you, I will rather think about the most impact you can make in the process. That is what ultimately replicates itself meaningfully in the numbers on your pay check, not just the expectation of Friday on Monday, at 9:00 am of the latter. Though this also may be a joke, yet carry a very interesting food for thought.

If you have even run a Bodega at the corner of a street, you will just talk less, about the nuances of business, a conglomerate that you probably know nothing about, than what you get on Friday; your pay check. It is not that money is the most important thing that keeps them awake at night, yet it is. They just respond to the dictates of the market place. This market place, have a lot of stake holders that include you and I.

The fundamentals of economics, give both the businesses and you some kind of leverage. The businesses though, just respond to our needs, judging from what we buy and use the most. If you think you want healthy food, and do not buy and use the most, and also if society preaches the benefits of healthy food as it related to your wellbeing and happiness, including good health itself, and you believe it and make the right choices or even demand it, I think McDonalds and the likes will adjust accordingly. The menus are not written in stone either. They change according to your needs, judging from your consumption habits. The next time we point the wrong finger at them, let's just remember the same finger we licked the last time. I think we all have a responsibility here.

All I am trying to say here is, the blame game is not the right way to go. The big question though is this. Will you produce something that no one will buy or has not shown much interest in buying? Why then do you want McDonalds to do so? The issue then is, we are all in it together. The entire chain of industrial, economic and socio-cultural and geo-political systems need a cautious but meaningful revamp. In addition any others that well permeate our life style have to merge, and revamp as well little by little with the goal of reaching a harmonized solution that make sense for everyone.

The returns on marketing dollars are the most inefficient business expenditures, yet you cannot do without it. To remake markets or fiddle with market shared at the speed of light, as we expect it will just not cut it. It will only work in the food industry, if we also can control your taste buds and change our habits at the same speed, with the creative collaboration of all related stakeholders.

Another joke. With all seriousness the dynamics of the market place as it relates to specific businesses or even an industry is not that simple to discern or pushed around as some may wish or even society as a whole. Sometimes it takes a lot of talent, team effort and fruitless cold cash to work, if you are even lucky.

Honestly, I think aside of the theories we learn in business school, the real business school, if you will call it a school, is on the stage, not necessary in the classroom, though that also helps. That is why we need this concept to at least, help in conjunction with others we know well already, to reach our expected systemic goals or improvements in our health, well being and ultimately happiness. By this concept, I mean "the systemic integrative thinking approach to problem solving". This will engender the requisite creative collaboration that will help foster the appropriate systemic changes needed in the entire ecosystem, toward the right equilibrium, or harmonized state.

If we are able to do that, the solutions coming out of the entire system, will definitely produce the appropriate expected outcomes, given our collective goals in mind. Though it is easier said that than, there is no other better alternative, if we are very serious about our set goals or expected benefits. To caution though, an iterative, and gradual systemic changes well thought out, with creative collaborative efforts of all, or at least most dominate stakeholders will get us there little by little, not at the speed of light as most of us would expect.

Satiety

At this point, I am going to talk a bit about the endocrine system, as it relates to Hunger. I will make it simple, but try my best to explain what was said by the researchers from the University of California, regarding the biochemical reason why we over eat.

Though I am going to talk about what pushed the thrust so fast after the 80' as it relates to the global demographics, it is not to blame anyone. Let us get into the science a bit, but not too much to again loose anyone. There is a hormone called Leptin. It somehow helps us to know that we are OK, and stop eating, at least too much. There is another called Peptide YY, which also signals to the brain that all the food we eat, has been fully digested and it is all clear in our waste pipe [Intestines].When they work well, you do not typically over eat.

They say some time after the 80', the industrial global diet, change our dietary patterns which promulgated, high sugar and carbohydrate intake which somehow, abnormally increased the insulin in our bodies. As I said before, if the quarter back does not work well, we lose the game.

Hence too much insulin causes leptin resistance, and other related problems for its contemporary, I just mentioned. Though a mouth full, it only means, it does not tell you the right time to stop eating, so you keep on eating. By the way, the global industrial diet, does not only come from fast foods. All other processed food is also part of it.

As I said before, it is very complex to even make a comment as a novice who have not ever run a bodega before. [A joke] I strongly believe, if they put the right people on the round table, they will eventually find at least a workable solution today, and a better tomorrow, and the next and the next. Though they may knock some heads, but that is OK. That in fact is how it is done everywhere. But it can be done. The diversity of interest will always play out. Yet if we understand that it is not a tag of war. We are all in a titanic sinking, and we will all go down, irrespective of the nature of our cabin. With that common understanding, the issue then for any reasonable person becomes how we save the titanic, so we all do not sink.

Not necessarily the soft cozy sofa in our cabin. For it may not make sense at the bottom of the ocean, or even makes a difference whether you had a cane chair or a leather sofa in your cabin. Or even a bunker bed.

The leptin theory, is one of the schools of thought which have created the requisite imbalance in our bodies energy regulatory systems, hence creating excess fat in our adipose tissue, by the process of adiposity, which eventually get us a little heavy setting, then obese and finally morbidly obese.

The imbalance also is fueled by our sedentary lifestyle. Those keep most of the fat or excess fat intact. If there is anything to blame here; it is a lot than can even write another book about. However I would simply say, the over leveraging of convenience in our society. Efficiency is great, but in the same vein, too much of everything is not good. We clamor for machine to do almost everything for as. Since the technology is there, someone will get it done and cash out, sometimes without close deep analysis of its impact, if not to society at large, for him, and children, and even children's children.

If we live an active life, or exercise more at least some of it will be shed. The question again then is, when we exercise or live active life, we get hungry again. Though we do, and eat, be cautious not to stuff in too much sugar, polish carbohydrates or too much of anything. Just keep them in wise moderation. When after exercising you drink too much sugar concentrated drinks, you only heighten your risk for leptin resistance, which is triggered by high insulin, which sugar or polished carbohydrates in excess are the main culprits.

I first talked about the market forces that regulated aggregate demand and supply, which kind of reaches equilibrium due to the tag of war between the flexing of muscles by the consumers and the producers or suppliers. Though the producers have a lot of marketing apparatus to flex their muscles, consumers may not have that per say individually, however, if they really are well educated about their needs, collectively as well as intensities of related risks, their power will be quite a formidable force in the market dynamics, if they use those information to make rational choices.

I do not and will not advocate any undue and unwarranted manipulation of the free market system. I think it can self regulate to a large extent, with the right structures in place. The only caveat is, on the consumer side; Are they well educated to make the right choices that will meet their apparent needs, which will ultimately improve their well being?

When I graduated from college, I quickly took the bus, which we called the Government Transport or The State Transport Corporation bus to my home town, which is called Kumasi in the Ashanti Region of Ghana. When I got home, my Dad was at the office. I then went to his factory to say hi. When I go there, he sat me down and we started charting. He then said congratulations, how was your finals. I said it all went well but we will see, though I know not all of them did.

Then he said, from what you learnt from school, tell me in a few words, what your understanding of Economics is. Armed with my fresh memory form the finals, I started quoting stuff from my text books here and there. He then said, Kwasi wait a minute. I said a few words, not a long story. In fact, I could not find words fewer than I was trying to. He then said, in it's simplest form, Economics is just how we manage our ends, to achieve our best well being and happiness. And that is all.

The question then is are the consumers armed with the information needed to manage their ultimate well being to the best of their ability, and is financially capable, by the choices they make in the market place. If they do, how do they react to demand it. I believe as I have said before, business plans are not written in stone, especially these days. Businesses only respond to our needs and wants, whatever shows up in their data. If I start getting into the various dynamics which we will have time to discuss a bit latter in volume two of this series, yet not in very much details, it will be clearer, that the blame game is just not the best way to solve any problem. Better collaborative team effort will serve us better.

The Reward Center of the Brain

Another factor I would like to talk about is the mechanism that creates human addiction which also perpetuates our unreasonable addiction to some kind of food items. There are some food groups deemed pleasure food. They are the likes of sugar sweets and other snacks made with carbohydrates that easily turn into sugar.

The over indulgence of these for any reason, creates a chronic stimulation of the sector of the brain that rewards us from eating such food item. The over stimulating however blunts the reward system of the brain so we even over indulge more, creating more problems related to obesity and its co-morbidities. (The bluntness of the reward system which is supposed to cause us to say enough is enough, is caused by the ill response of dopamine and fuel receptors – which then leads to addiction to these substances; sugar, salt, cabs all of which have a negative impact on metabolic syndrome and the other problems we talked about earlier. I am not saying no one should eat potato chip, because I do. I am only suggesting that we do these things with moderate caution.

Too much of everything is bad, so is too much of nothing. A little stimulation of the Nucleus Accumben is OK. Though over stimulation of it, can get you addicted to anything, from coffee to sugar, salt and so on. The name I threw out is not to scare anyone, since I know it is a mouth full. It is simply the brains reward center, which influences our propensity or inclination for addiction, if we over indulge in anything with such potentials.

Genetic Predispositions

Genetics is another factor that affects our fate with obesity. Just as we do not choose our parents, there is not much to do here. I know I cannot do much about my UGLY nose. Even if I had the money, plastic surgery cannot change my face much. Yet when I look in the mirror, the combination of all that is in my face makes me feel that God made me just fine.

All I am saying here is that, you may not be able to do much about your genetic predispositions. You can fuss with your nose and mouth or whatever, though the hair is an exception, you are simply stuck with them. If you look closely though, it fit in with the rest beautifully.

Another important point about genetics which brought up all this is that, if you are predisposed to be obese or even have cancer, though you are stuck with it, it does not necessarily mean you will get it. Their manifestation has a lot to do also with the way we live our lives and the choices we make, coupled with other environmental factors.

Some of these choices, especially regarding professional and work environments, you personally may not have much leverage in the choices that are made, or you may if you happen to be the boss. Yet there are a lot of choices in life that are within our control. As to having the will power, and right information to make the right choices is very totally up to you, though not absolutely, especially if you are fully aware of the health risk factors and their environmental carcinogens or triggers.

I however also threw in "not absolutely" to throw in a caveat. It is simply because sometimes we are stuck with the choices in front of us in the market of proximity, which leaves a little room to make appropriate choices.

For example, if you know your parents had diabetes, and you drink alcohol excessively which gravitates into an addiction, which blinds your capacity to resist irrespective of its apparent health risks to you. Then who do you blame? Not that I may not empathize with you for your pain, since we are all not perfect, there is no one to blame.

Another very important factor that I will talk about briefly, though I have already, is again genetics. It is important that in the nearest future, we make an effort to understand the fate our genome affords us. As I said before, you are stuck with, whether you know or not. It may be still good to know; especially if it gives enough education about YOU, in relation to your health and well being in general. The relevance of this though is so you make the appropriate choices that will help you to prevent, issues that can possibly make you unhappy, sick and even disabled and poor.

Sometimes most of all these outcomes can be prevented, if you are aware of the apparent consequences. In fact, it can help you make the appropriate life style choices that will probably give you enough time to pay off your lay away

" " till your final time is up. You can also enjoy life more with your family or by yourself, depending on what you choose, in a very healthy body. Rather than with a ton of aches and pains that could have been avoided. The good news though is what it takes to know is already here. May be, not in my hometown in Kumasi, though I know eventually it will get there too. But there is no excuse for anyone who live between LA and NY either than money to complain to not know. We will end the genetics talk here.

Chronic Stress

Stress is another main factor which fuels our propensities toward being obese. It is though a normal reaction in animals or humans in particular which help us to avoid danger. There is a hormone called cortical which regulate our level of stress. Though I say it is good, too much of it could cause you to be hungry and eat too much or cause other metabolic dysfunctions that can affect your health in general.

It is not something that has to be a perpetual response, since we do not face dangers everyday in our lives. Unfortunately the dangers that our forefathers, the CAVE MEN faced were wild animals. Their reaction to stress was predicated by how fast you could run away. Today, thing have changed, yet for the better or worse, what it is, is what it is. Our lives or good segment of our demographic are constantly afraid. We are afraid of almost everything including sometimes our own shadow which does not even have the capacity to bite or even harm in anyway.

In the medical field, we call it environmental chronic stress. We again will have the chance to talk about it later in a little detail in the next volume of this series. I will at least attempt to identify some of the triggers of environmental chronic stress that is making us all afraid most of the time, of practically nothing.

As a result of these kinds of environmental stressors and their impact on the body, we tend to eat more because we get hungry more and crave for calories, traditionally to help us run faster away from the wild animals. You and I know the closest zoo perhaps is miles away and even then, we go there to have fun, because all the wild animals are all caged. What is the purpose of the craving for excessive calories to help us run faster? The answer though is that, we have not changed much in terms of our human physiology as it relates to these mechanisms. We are still designed to run away as the CAVE MEN did, though this time funny enough, from our own imaginations or shadows.

This though may sound funny; there are sometimes threats that are eminent, especially those that sometime threaten our economic stability. Even here, most of them are initiated with rumors that often turn out hot air.

Some from the remotest areas in Africa learn about tigers and lion from text books. All I am saying is that if you have a safe conscience, even if not perfect, there is no need to be afraid, or invoke the mechanism to run, by rushing cortisol through you at risky perpetual levels.

It is just a survival mechanism that has unfortunately become a way of life. I would say though that there is a better life, if you want to know, though it is not appropriate to say it here. Therefore I will leave it up to you to find what is best for you. Most stressors are psychological with no rational tenets. Just like running away from our own shadow which only stops when you do.

Voluntary or involuntary, stress could be minimized or controlled better with exercise, mindfulness practices, prayer and meditation. Or taking pragmatic steps to eliminate apparent risks even if they are real and apparent, especially related to means of livelihood. I may recommend that you do those more instead of just eating. Increasing your level of activity even slightly will help or go a long way.

For most men, our bellies are so bulgy. Some parts of the world, it was deemed a status symbol in the past. But I do not think that is the case today. Stress has a lot to do with it. When your stomach start bulging out, please act quickly, right on the onset, and hold the bull by the horn, because, I do not have too many friends, especially lady friends, who are enthused by the size of our belly. The pocket to some of them may compensate, yet over compensation with that, will raise a question. That is, if love have anything to do with the relationship.

At least Barbara did not fancy that, though Sweve scored lots of points. I may say it did not help much in his position in the queue, what I can say though is that, he was an excellent POLO Player, and did very well on his saddles. I may also say that he was quite as fit as a fiddle. Remember my study mate in Logon I told you about from the beginning. I hope you take this as another joke brake, till be get more serious again.

The Pathogenesis of Metabolic Syndrome and Related Issues and definitions

This heading may be a mouth full again. Yet it simply means the beginning of the formation of metabolic syndrome and related health indications. It is very hard to explain these complex phenomena in simple terms. As I have already mentioned before, our friends at Wiki always saves the day. They somehow have a good knack for demystifying myths in complex phenomena or processes in very simple terms. Again, this is not an advertisement for Wiki, yet I honestly cannot do it better.

I will therefore, pick a few articles from Wiki, that explains most of the related complex phenomena that interactively and single handedly causes such indications to emerge as a result of metabolic syndrome.

We will therefore start with Hypertension. In simple terms, it is when the cardio vascular system works too hard than normal to circulate blood or to pump blood through the body to feed the various cells with the needed nutrient or ingredient needed for them to perform their respective functions. Such ingredients or nutrients as oxygen, vitamins, water and so on, are transported to the entire body for the various subsystems to function well to keep a person healthy and going.

The heart is what filters and pump the blood. The used blood returns to the heart, get cleaned and get passed along again. The lungs add oxygen to it, and on it goes. This process is one of the most essential pieces of work that life depends on. Without blood flowing normally lots of problems can occur inhibiting normal development, and functioning of the body.

The pipes that carry the blood through the body are the veins and arteries. The difference between them is simply, who take the clean blood to the organs and who carry the dirty or used to the heart. The free flow of blood in and out of the heart is equally essential to healthy living, and proper functioning of our body. It is also very critical to life itself.

Unfortunately, when one does not eat properly or have some genetic characteristics that make the body prone to such issues as we are going to describe, and also for other reasons, some plague gradually start forming from the residue of some bad nutrients which with time, sometimes a very long time, thickens the walls of these arteries and veins, inhibiting the flexibility of these pipes that carries blood through the body.

In its worse forms, it makes them difficult to normally expand and contract in a way that makes the work of the heart gets a bit difficult. When it gets very hard, it takes too much work for the blood to be pushed through easily as it normally should for some reasons, two of which are most critical. The first one is, the plaques make the area circumference smaller. It can then be inferred that, less blood can pass through them normally.

Since the heart therefore do not slow its rhythm to accommodate the reduction in the size of the pipe. You can then imagine how frustrated it would be. I would draw a similar synergy in computer networking for those of you who are a bit technologically savvy. When a relatively large amount of data is push through a pipe with a small bandwidth, what is going to happen?

The least will, be complications in invocation of the protocol mechanisms that resend dropped packets due to the congestion and related handshakes by the end nodes. This obviously can cause some tardiness in respective applications that follow that path.

The issue I am trying to highlight here is that, when a pipe gets smaller than the needed traffic that has to go through it, there are always problems obviously. A traffic jam from a road construction can also be a good example which most of us can relate to. If it does nothing to you, just check your blood pressure in a traffic jam, when you are already late to work.

The other issue is, the inflexibility, due to the thickening of the walls. This also inhibits it from expanding appropriately to accommodate, the volume of blood as it would normally. For some of you who have a bit of physics in your blood and especially a little savvy with issues relating to the flow of fluids, you will bear with me that, viscosity is another issue that affects the free flow of fluids.

Viscosity is however, well influenced by the density of the fluid. I hope Mr. Owusu Mensah will be proud of me after all. Since he was my last formal physics teacher. At least he did not waste his time with me, though it has taken too long to use this aspect of what he thought me, at least in my writings. The most I think he will be proud of, is advising me to take the healthcare position in high school, which has of late heightened my passion again, especially relating to the Obesity Epidemic and related issues. I will therefore say thanks again before I move on. Because you said, if I do not take it I may regret in the future. I have come to appreciate your advice, because I will have really missed out.

This then bring us to the third issue with blood flow through the body. This issue is exacerbated by salt content of the food we eat. It also affects the ease with which blood travels back and forth throw cell membranes to deliver its goodies. I am not going to explain osmosis and the other related phenomena, to turn this into a biology class. I know my biology teacher, "Expensive" as we used to call him, is alive, but I will not let him rival my old friend, Mr. Owusu Mensah, hence will end the biology here. For those of you who care a bit for a little more insight, I will leave you with the following article from Wiki:

"Atherosclerosis (also known as arteriosclerotic vascular disease or ASVD) is a specific form of arteriosclerosis in which an artery wall thickens as a result of the accumulation of calcium and fatty materials such as cholesterol and triglyceride. It reduces the elasticity of the artery walls and therefore allows less blood to travel through. This also increases blood pressure. It is a syndrome affecting arterial blood vessels, a chronic inflammatory response in the walls of arteries, caused largely by the accumulation of macrophages and white blood cells and promoted by low-density lipoproteins (LDL, plasma proteins that carry cholesterol and triglycerides) without adequate removal of fats and cholesterol from the macrophages by functional high-density lipoproteins (HDL) (see apoA-1 Milano). It is commonly referred to as a hardening or furring of the arteries. It is caused by the formation of multiple plaques within the arteries. The atheromatous plaque is divided into three distinct components:

1. The atheroma ("lump of gruel", from Greek (athera), meaning "gruel"), which is the nodular accumulation of a soft, flaky, yellowish material at the center of large plaques, composed of macrophages nearest the lumen of the artery
2. Underlying areas of cholesterol crystals
3. Calcification at the outer base of older/more advanced lesions.

The following terms are similar, yet distinct, in both spelling and meaning, and can be easily confused: arteriosclerosis, arteriolosclerosis, and atherosclerosis. Arteriosclerosis is a general term describing any hardening (and loss of elasticity) of medium or large arteries (from Greek (artria), meaning "artery", and (sklerosis), meaning "hardening"); arteriolosclerosis is any hardening (and loss of elasticity) of arterioles (small arteries); atherosclerosis is a hardening of an artery specifically due to an atheromatous plaque. The term atherogenic is used for substances or processes that cause atherosclerosis.[citation needed]

Atherosclerosis is a chronic disease that remains asymptomatic for decades. Atherosclerotic lesions, or atherosclerotic plaques are separated into two broad categories: Stable and unstable (also called vulnerable). The pathobiology of atherosclerotic lesions is very complicated but generally, stable atherosclerotic plaques, which tend to be asymptomatic, are rich in extracellular matrix and smooth muscle cells, while, unstable plaques are rich in macrophages and foam cells and the extracellular matrix separating the lesion from the arterial lumen (also known as the fibrous cap) is usually weak and prone to rupture. Ruptures of the fibrous cap expose thrombogenic material, such as collagen to the circulation and eventually induce thrombus formation in the lumen. Upon formation, intraluminal thrombi can occlude arteries outright (e.g. coronary occlusion), but more often they detach, move into the circulation and eventually occluding smaller downstream branches causing thromboembolism. Apart from thromboembolism, chronically expanding atherosclerotic lesions can cause complete closure of the lumen. Interestingly, chronically expanding lesions are often asymptomatic until lumen stenosis is so severe (usually over 80%) that blood supply to downstream tissue(s) is insufficient, resulting in ischemia.

These complications of advanced atherosclerosis are chronic, slowly progressive and cumulative. Most commonly, soft plaque suddenly ruptures (see vulnerable plaque), causing the formation of a thrombus that will rapidly slow or stop blood flow, leading to death of the tissues fed by the artery in approximately 5 minutes. This catastrophic event is called an infarction. One of the most common recognized scenarios is called coronary thrombosis of a coronary artery, causing myocardial infarction (a heart attack). The same process in an artery to the brain is commonly called stroke. Another common scenario in very advanced disease is claudication from insufficient blood supply to the legs, typically caused by a combination of both stenosis and aneurysmal segments narrowed with clots.

Atherosclerosis affects the entire artery tree, but mostly larger, high-pressure vessels such as the coronary, renal, femoral, cerebral, and carotid arteries. These are termed "clinically silent" because the person having the infarction does not notice the problem and does not seek medical help, or when they do, physicians do not recognize what has happened.

Signs and symptoms

Atherosclerosis is often asymptomatic pending grave blockage and narrowing of an artery. Signs and symptoms usually come out when the severe blockage impedes blood flow to different organs. Most of the time, patients realize that they have the disease only when they experience other cardio vascular disorders such as stroke or heart attack. These symptoms, however, still vary depending on which artery or organ is affected. Typically, atherosclerosis begins as a thin layer of white streaks on the artery wall (usually due to white blood cells) and progresses from there. Clinically, atherosclerosis is typically associated with men over the age of 45. Sub-clinically, the disease begins to appear at early childhood, and perhaps even at birth. Noticeable signs can begin developing at puberty. Though symptoms are rarely exhibited in children, early screening of children for cardiovascular diseases could be beneficial to both the child and his/her relatives. While coronary artery disease is more prevalent in men than women, atherosclerosis of the cerebral arteries and strokes equally affect both sexes.

Blockage in the coronary arteries, which are responsible for bringing oxygenated blood to the heart, can have symptoms such as chest pain of angina and shortness of breath, sweating, nausea, dizziness or light-headedness, breathlessness or palpitations. Abnormal heart rhythms called arrhythmias, where the heart is either beating too slow or too fast, is also considered a symptom. Carotid arteries are used to supply blood to the brain and neck. Blockage in them present symptoms such as a feeling of weakness, not being able to think straight, difficulty in speaking, being dizzy and difficulty in walking or standing up straight, blurred vision, numbness of the face, arms, and legs, severe headache and losing consciousness. These symptoms are also related to stroke. Stroke is caused by blockage of majority arteries going to the brain where lack of oxygen will lead to the death of the cells of the affected tissue. Peripheral arteries, which supply blood to the legs, arms, and pelvis, could also experience blockage due to plaque formation. Symptoms for the blockage here are numbness to the arms or legs, as well at pain. Another significant location for the plaque formation are the renal arteries, which would supply blood to the kidneys. Plaque occurrence and accumulation here could lead to chronic kidney disease, which are asymptomatic at its early stage.

Causes

The atherosclerotic process is not fully understood. Atherosclerosis is initiated by inflammatory processes in the endothelial cells of the vessel wall in response to retained low-density lipoprotein (LDL) molecules.

Lipoproteins in the blood vary in size. Some data suggests that only small dense LDL (sdLDL) particles are able to get behind the cellular monolayer of endothelium. LDL particles and their content are susceptible to oxidation by free radicals, and the risk may be higher while in the bloodstream. However, LDL particles have a half-life of only a couple of days, and their content (LDL particles carry cholesterol, cholesteryl esters, and tryglycerides from the liver to the tissues of the body) changes with time.

Once inside the vessel wall, LDL particles get stuck and their content becomes more prone to oxidation. The damage caused by the oxidized LDL molecules triggers a cascade of immune responses which over time can produce an atheroma. First the immune system sends specialized white blood cells (macrophages and T-lymphocytes) to absorb the oxidized LDL, forming specialized foam cells. These white blood cells are not able to process the oxidized LDL. They grow and then rupture, depositing a greater amount of oxidized cholesterol into the artery wall. This triggers more white blood cells, continuing the cycle. Eventually, the artery becomes inflamed. The cholesterol plaque causes the muscle cells to enlarge and form a hard cover over the affected area. This hard cover is what causes a narrowing of the artery, reducing blood flow and increasing blood pressure.

Some researchers believe that atherosclerosis may be caused by an infection of the vascular smooth muscle cells. Chickens, for example, develop atherosclerosis when infected with the Marek's disease herpesvirus. Herpesvirus infection of arterial smooth muscle cells has been shown to cause cholesteryl ester (CE) accumulation, which is associated with atherosclerosis. Cytomegalovirus

(CMV) infection is also associated with cardiovascular diseases.

Risk factors

Various anatomic and physiological risk factors for atherosclerosis are known. These can be divided into various categories: congenital vs acquired, modifiable or not, classical or non-classical. The points labelled '+' in the following list form the core components of metabolic syndrome.

Risks multiply, with two factors increasing the risk of atherosclerosis fourfold. Hyperlipidemia, hypertension and cigarette smoking together increases the risk seven times.

Dietary

The relation between dietary fat and atherosclerosis is a contentious field. The USDA, in its food pyramid, promotes a low-fat diet, based largely on its view that fat in the diet is atherogenic. The American Heart Association, the American Diabetes Association and the National Cholesterol Education Program make similar recommendations. In contrast, Prof Walter Willett (Harvard School of Public Health, PI of the second Nurses' Health Study) recommends much higher levels, especially of monounsaturated and polyunsaturated fat. Writing in Science, Gary Taubes detailed that political considerations played into the recommendations of government bodies.

These differing views reach a consensus, though, against consumption of trans fats. The role of dietary oxidized fats/lipid peroxidation (rancid fats) in humans is not clear. Laboratory animals fed rancid fats develop atherosclerosis. Rats fed DHA-containing oils experienced marked disruptions to their antioxidant systems, and accumulated significant amounts of phospholipid hydroperoxide in their blood, livers and kidneys. I n another study, rabbits fed atherogenic diets containing various oils were found to undergo the greatest amount of oxidative susceptibility of LDL via polyunsaturated oils. In a study involving rabbits fed heated soybean oil, "grossly induced atherosclerosis and marked liver damage were histologically and clinically demonstrated." However,

Kummerow, a prominent researcher, claims that it is not dietary cholesterol, but oxysterols, or oxidized cholesterols, from fried foods and smoking, that are the culprit.

Rancid fats and oils taste very bad even in small amounts, so people avoid eating them. It is very difficult to measure or estimate the actual human consumption of these substances.

Highly unsaturated omega-3 rich oils such as fish oil are being sold in pill form so that the taste of oxidized or rancid fat is not apparent. The health food industry's dietary supplements are self regulated by the manufacture and outside of FDA regulations. To properly protect unsaturated fats from oxidation, it is best to keep them cool and in oxygen free environments. Long term exposure to inorganic arsenic can cause atherosclerosis.

Pathophysiology

Atherogenesis is the developmental process of atheromatous plaques. It is characterized by a remodeling of arteries leading to subendothelial accumulation of fatty substances called plaques. The build up of an atheromatous plaque is a slow process, developed over a period of several years through a complex series of cellular events occurring within the arterial wall, and in response to a variety of local vascular circulating factors. One recent hypothesis suggests that, for unknown reasons, leukocytes, such as monocytes or basophils, begin to attack the endothelium of the artery lumen in cardiac muscle. The ensuing inflammation leads to formation of atheromatous plaques in the arterial tunica intima, a region of the vessel wall located between the endothelium and the tunica media. The bulk of these lesions is made of excess fat, collagen, and elastin. At first, as the plaques grow, only wall thickening occurs without any narrowing. Stenosis is a late event, which may never occur and is often the result of repeated plaque rupture and healing responses, not just the atherosclerotic process by itself.

Cellular

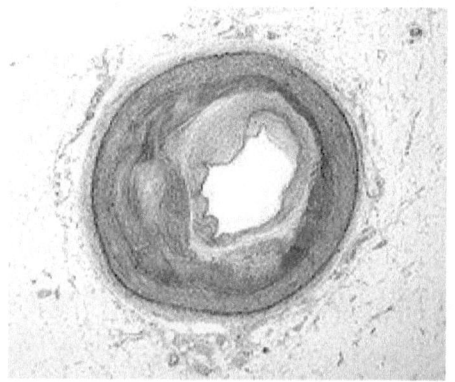

Micrograph of an artery that supplies the heart showing significant atherosclerosis and marked luminal narrowing. Tissue has been stained using Masson's trichrome.

Early atherogenesis is characterized by the adherence of blood circulating monocytes (a type of white blood cell) to the vascular bed lining, the endothelium, followed by their migration to the sub-endothelial space, and further activation into monocyte-derived macrophages. The primary documented driver of this process is oxidized lipoprotein particles within the wall, beneath the endothelial cells, though upper normal or elevated concentrations of blood glucose also plays a major role and not all factors are fully understood. Fatty streaks may appear and disappear.

Low-density lipoprotein (LDL) particles in blood plasma invade the endothelium and become oxidized, creating risk of cardiovascular disease. A complex set of biochemical reactions regulates the oxidation of LDL, involving enzymes (such as Lp-LpA2) and free radicals in the endothelium.

Initial damage to the endothelium results in an inflammatory response. Monocytes enter the artery wall from the bloodstream, with platelets adhering to the area of insult. This may be promoted by redox signaling induction of factors such as VCAM-1, which recruit circulating monocytes, and M-CSF, which is selectively required for the differentiation of monocytes to macrophages. The monocytes differentiate into macrophages, which ingest oxidized LDL, slowly turning into large "foam cells" –

so-called because of their changed appearance resulting from the numerous internal cytoplasmic vesicles and resulting high lipid content. Under the microscope, the lesion now appears as a fatty streak. Foam cells eventually die, and further propagate the inflammatory process. There is also smooth muscle proliferation and migration from the tunica media into the intima responding to cytokines secreted by damaged endothelial cells. This causes the formation of a fibrous capsule covering the fatty streak. Intact endothelium could prevent the proliferation by releasing nitric oxide.

Calcification and lipids

Calcification forms among vascular smooth muscle cells of the surrounding muscular layer, specifically in the muscle cells adjacent to atheromas and on the surface of atheroma plaques and tissue. In time, as cells die, this leads to extracellular calcium deposits between the muscular wall and outer portion of the atheromatous plaques. With the atheromatous plaque interfering with the regulation of the calcium deposition, it accumulates and crystallizes. A similar form of an intramural calcification, presenting the picture of an early phase of arteriosclerosis, appears to be induced by a number of drugs that have an antiproliferative mechanism of action (Rainer Liedtke 2008).

Cholesterol is delivered into the vessel wall by cholesterol-containing low-density lipoprotein (LDL) particles. To attract and stimulate macrophages, the cholesterol must be released from the LDL particles and oxidized, a key step in the ongoing inflammatory process. The process is worsened if there is insufficient high-density lipoprotein (HDL), the lipoprotein particle that removes cholesterol from tissues and carries it back to the liver.

The foam cells and platelets encourage the migration and proliferation of smooth muscle cells, which in turn ingest lipids, become replaced by collagen and transform into foam cells themselves. A protective fibrous cap normally forms between the fatty deposits and the artery lining (the intima).

These capped fatty deposits (now called 'atheromas') produce enzymes that cause the artery to enlarge over time. As long as the artery enlarges sufficiently to compensate for the extra thickness of the atheroma, then no narrowing ("stenosis") of the opening ("lumen") occurs. The artery becomes expanded with an egg-shaped cross-section, still with a circular opening. If the enlargement is beyond proportion to the atheroma thickness, then an aneurysm is created.[50]

Visible features

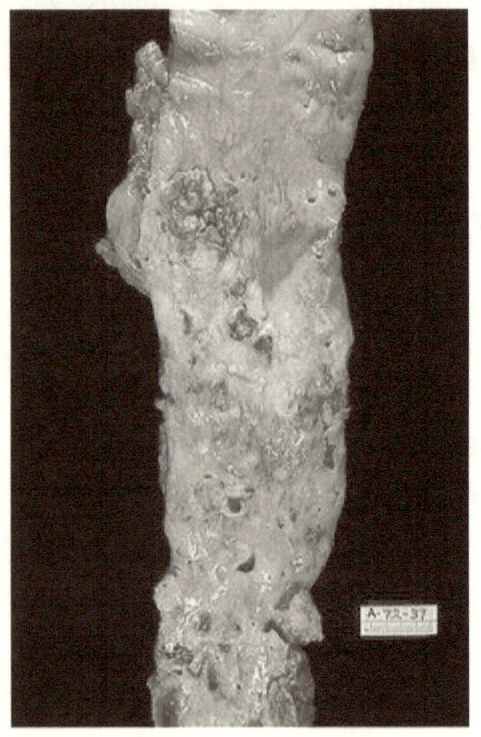

Severe atherosclerosis of the aorta. Autopsy specimen. Although arteries are not typically studied microscopically, two plaque types can be distinguished.

The fibro-lipid (fibro-fatty) plaque is characterized by an accumulation of lipid-laden cells underneath the intima of the arteries, typically without narrowing the lumen due to compensatory expansion of the bounding muscular layer of the artery wall. Beneath the endothelium there is a "fibrous cap" covering the atheromatous "core" of the plaque. The core consists of lipid-laden cells (macrophages and smooth muscle cells) with elevated tissue cholesterol and cholesterol ester content, fibrin, proteoglycans, collagen, elastin, and cellular debris. In advanced plaques, the central core of the plaque usually contains extracellular cholesterol deposits (released from dead cells), which form areas of cholesterol crystals with empty, needle-like clefts. At the periphery of the plaque are younger "foamy" cells and capillaries. These plaques usually produce the most damage to the individual when they rupture.

The fibrous plaque is also localized under the intima, within the wall of the artery resulting in thickening and expansion of the wall and, sometimes, spotty localized narrowing of the lumen with some atrophy of the muscular layer. The fibrous plaque contains collagen fibers (eosinophilic), precipitates of calcium (hematoxylinophilic) and, rarely, lipid-laden cells.

In effect, the muscular portion of the artery wall forms small aneurysms just large enough to hold the atheroma that are present. The muscular portion of artery walls usually remain strong, even after they have remodeled to compensate for the atheromatous plaques.

However, atheromas within the vessel wall are soft and fragile with little elasticity. Arteries constantly expand and contract with each heartbeat, i.e., the pulse. In addition, the calcification deposits between the outer portion of the atheroma and the muscular wall, as they progress, lead to a loss of elasticity and stiffening of the artery as a whole.

The calcification deposits, after they have become sufficiently advanced, are partially visible on coronary artery computed tomography or electron beam tomography (EBT) as rings of increased radiographic density, forming halos around the outer edges of the atheromatous plaques, within the artery wall. On CT, >130 units on the Hounsfield scale (some argue for 90 units) has been the radiographic density usually accepted as clearly representing tissue calcification within arteries. These deposits demonstrate unequivocal evidence of the disease, relatively advanced, even though the lumen of the artery is often still normal by angiographic or intravascular ultrasound.

Rupture and stenosis

Although the disease process tends to be slowly progressive over decades, it usually remains asymptomatic until an atheroma ulcerates, which leads to immediate blood clotting at the site of atheroma ulcer. This triggers a cascade of events that leads to clot enlargement, which may quickly obstruct the flow of blood. A complete blockage leads to ischemia of the myocardial (heart) muscle and damage. This process is the myocardial infarction or "heart attack".

If the heart attack is not fatal, fibrous organization of the clot within the lumen ensues, covering the rupture but also producing stenosis or closure of the lumen, or over time and after repeated ruptures, resulting in a persistent, usually localized stenosis or blockage of the artery lumen. Stenoses can be slowly progressive, whereas plaque ulceration is a sudden event that occurs specifically in atheromas with thinner/weaker fibrous caps that have become "unstable".

Repeated plaque ruptures, ones not resulting in total lumen closure, combined with the clot patch over the rupture and healing response to stabilize the clot, is the process that produces most stenoses over time. The stenotic areas tend to become more stable, despite increased flow velocities at these narrowings. Most major blood-flow-stopping events occur at large plaques, which, prior to their rupture, produced very little if any stenosis.

From clinical trials, 20% is the average stenosis at plaques that subsequently rupture with resulting complete artery closure. Most severe clinical events do not occur at plaques that produce high-grade stenosis. From clinical trials, only 14% of heart attacks occur from artery closure at plaques producing a 75% or greater stenosis prior to the vessel closing.[citation needed]

If the fibrous cap separating a soft atheroma from the bloodstream within the artery ruptures, tissue fragments are exposed and released. These tissue fragments are very clot-promoting, containing collagen and tissue factor; they activate platelets and activate the system of coagulation. The result is the formation of a thrombus (blood clot) overlying the atheroma, which obstructs blood flow acutely. With the obstruction of blood flow, downstream tissues are starved of oxygen and nutrients. If this is the myocardium (heart muscle), angina (cardiac chest pain) or myocardial infarction (heart attack) develops.

Diagnosis

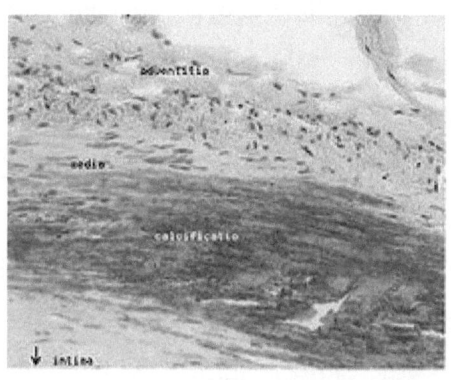

Microphotography of arterial wall with calcified (violet colour) atherosclerotic plaque (haematoxillin & eosin stain)

Areas of severe narrowing, stenosis, detectable by angiography, and to a lesser extent "stress testing" have long been the focus of human diagnostic techniques for cardiovascular disease, in general. However, these methods focus on detecting only severe narrowing, not the underlying atherosclerosis disease. As demonstrated by human clinical studies, most severe events occur in locations with heavy plaque, yet little or no lumen narrowing present before debilitating events suddenly occur. Plaque rupture can lead to artery lumen occlusion within seconds to minutes, and potential permanent debility and sometimes sudden death.

Plaques that have ruptured are called complicated plaques. The extracellular matrix of the lesion breaks, usually at the shoulder of the fibrous cap that separates the lesion from the arterial lumen, where the exposed thrombogenic components of the plaque, mainly collagen will trigger thrombus formation. The thrombus then travel downstream to other blood vessels, where the blood clot may partially or completely block blood flow. If the blood flow is completely blocked, cell deaths occur due to the lack of oxygen supply to nearby cells, resulting in necrosis. The narrowing or obstruction of blood flow can occur in any artery within the body. Obstruction of arteries supplying the heart muscle result in a heart attack, while the obstruction of arteries supplying the brain result in a stroke.

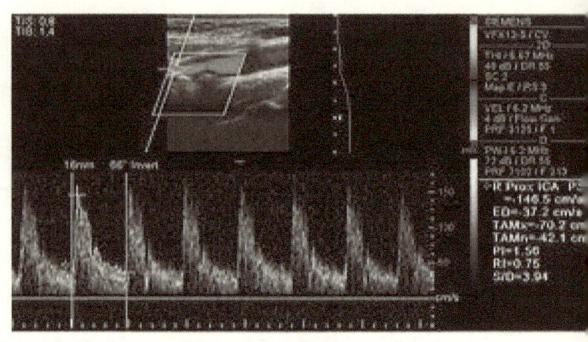

Doppler ultrasound of right internal Carotid artery with calcified and non-calcified plaques showing less than 70% stenosis

Lumen stenosis that is greater than 75% were considered as the hallmark of clinically significant disease in the past because recurring episodes of angina and abnormalities in stress test are only detectable at that particular severity of stenosis. However, clinical trials have shown that only about 14% of clinically debilitating events occur at sites with >75% stenosis. Majority of cardiovascular events that involve sudden rupture of the atheroma plaque do not display any evident narrowing of the lumen. Thus, greater attention has been focused on "vulnerable plaque" from the late 1990s onwards.

Besides the traditional diagnostic methods such as angiography and stress-testing, other detection techniques have been developed in the past decades for earlier detection of atherosclerotic disease. Some of the detection approaches include anatomical detection and physiologic measurement.

Examples of anatomical detection methods include coronary calcium scoring by CT, carotid IMT intimal media thickness measurement by ultrasound, and intravascular ultrasound (IVUS). Examples of physiologic measurement methods include lipoprotein subclass analysis, HbA1c, hs-CRP, and homocysteine. Both anatomic and physiologic methods allow early detection before symptoms show up, disease staging and tracking of disease progression. Anatomic methods are more expensive and some of them are invasive in nature, such as IVUS. On the other hand, physiologic methods are often less expensive and safer. But they do not quantify the current state of the disease or directly track progression. In the recent years, ways of estimating the severity of atherosclerotic plaques is also made possible with the developments in nuclear imaging techniques such as PET and SPECT.

Prevention

Combinations of statins, niacin, intestinal cholesterol absorption-inhibiting supplements (ezetimibe and others, and to a much lesser extent fibrates) have been the most successful in changing common but sub-optimal lipoprotein patterns and group outcomes. In the many secondary prevention and several primary prevention trials, several classes of lipoprotein-expression-altering (less correctly termed "cholesterol-lowering") agents have consistently reduced not only heart attack, stroke and hospitalization but also all-cause mortality rates. The first of the large secondary prevention comparative statin/placebo treatment trials was the Scandinavian Simvastatin Survival Study (4S) with over fifteen more studies extending through to the more recent ASTEROID trial published in 2006. The first primary prevention comparative treatment trial was AFCAPS/TexCAPS with multiple later comparative statin/placebo treatment trials including EXCEL, ASCOT and SPARCL. While the statin trials have all been clearly favorable for improved human outcomes, only ASTEROID and SATURN showed evidence of atherosclerotic regression (slight). Both human and animal trials that showed evidence of disease regression used more aggressive combination agent treatment strategies, which nearly always included niacin.

Treatment

Medical treatments often focus on alleviating symptoms. However measures which focus on decreasing underlying atherosclerosis—as opposed to simply treating symptoms—are more effective. Non-pharmaceutical means are usually the first method of treatment, such as stopping smoking and practicing regular exercise. If these methods do not work, medicines are usually the next step in treating cardiovascular diseases, and, with improvements, have increasingly become the most effective method over the long term.

The key to the more effective approaches has been better understanding of the widespread and insidious nature of the disease and to combine multiple different treatment strategies, not rely on just one or a few approaches. In addition, for those approaches, such as lipoprotein transport behaviors, which have been shown to produce the most success, adopting more aggressive combination treatment strategies taken on a daily basis and indefinitely has generally produced better results, both before and especially after people are symptomatic.

Statins

The group of medications referred to as statins are widely prescribed for treating atherosclerosis. They shown benefit in reducing cardiovascular disease and mortality in those with high cholesterol with few side effects. This data is primarily in middle-age men and the conclusions are less clear for women and people over the age of 70. Monocyte counts, as well as cholesterol markers such as LDL:HDL ratio and apolipiprotein B: apolipoprotein A-1 ratio can be used as markers to monitor the extent of atherosclerotic regression which proves useful in guiding patient treatments.

Diet

Changes in diet may help prevent the development of atherosclerosis.

Surgery

Other physical treatments, include angioplasty procedures that may include stents and bypass surgery.

Other

There is recent evidence that some anticoagulants, particularly warfarin, which inhibit clot formation by interfering with Vitamin K metabolism, may actually promote arterial calcification in the long term despite reducing clot formation in the short term.

Prognosis

Lipoprotein imbalances, upper normal and especially elevated blood sugar, i.e., diabetes and high blood pressure are risk factors for atherosclerosis; homocysteine, stopping smoking, taking anticoagulants (anti-clotting agents), which target clotting factors, taking omega-3 oils from fatty fish or plant oils such as flax or canola oils, exercising and losing weight are the usual focus of treatments that have proven to be helpful in clinical trials. The target serum cholesterol level should ideally not exceed 4 mmol/L (160 mg/dL), and triglycerides should not exceed 2 mmol/L (180 mg/dL).

Evidence has increased that diabetics, despite not having clinically detectable atherosclerotic disease, have more severe debility from atherosclerotic events over time than even non-diabetics who have already suffered atherosclerotic events. Thus diabetes has been upgraded to be viewed as an advanced atherosclerotic disease equivalent[clarification needed].

Research

An indication of the role of HDL on atherosclerosis has been with the rare Apo-Al Milano human genetic variant of this HDL protein. A small short-term trial using bacterial synthetized human Apo-Al Milano HDL in people with unstable angina produced fairly dramatic reduction in measured coronary plaque volume in only 6 weeks vs. the usual increase in plaque volume in those randomized to placebo. The trial was published in JAMA in early 2006. Ongoing work starting in the 1990s may lead to human clinical trials— probably by about 2008. These may use synthesized Apo-AI Milano HDL directly. Or they may use gene-transfer methods to pass the ability to synthesize the Apo-AI Milano HDLipoprotein.

Methods to increase high-density lipoprotein (HDL) particle concentrations, which in some animal studies largely reverses and remove atheromas, are being developed and researched.

Niacin has HDL raising effects (by 10-30%) and showed clinical trial benefit in the Coronary Drug Project and is commonly used in combination with other lipoprotein agents to improve efficacy of changing lipoprotein for the better. However most individuals have nuisance symptoms with short term flushing reactions, especially initially, and so working with a physician with a history of successful experience with niacin implementation, careful selection of brand, dosing strategy, etc. are usually critical to success.

However, increasing HDL by any means is not necessarily helpful. For example, the drug torcetrapib is the most effective agent currently known for raising HDL (by up to 60%). However, in clinical trials it also raised deaths by 60%. All studies regarding this drug were halted in December 2006. See CETP inhibitor for similar approaches.

The actions of macrophages drive atherosclerotic plaque progression. Immunomodulation of atherosclerosis is the term for techniques that modulate immune system function to suppress this macrophage action. Research on genetic expression and control mechanisms is progressing. Topics include PPAR, known to be important in blood sugar and variants of lipoprotein production and function;

The multiple variants of the proteins that form the lipoprotein transport particles. Some controversial research has suggested a link between atherosclerosis and the presence of several different nanobacteria in the arteries, e.g., Chlamydophila pneumoniae, though trials of current antibiotic treatments known to be usually effective in suppressing growth or killing these bacteria have not been successful in improving outcomes.

The immunomodulation approaches mentioned above, because they deal with innate responses of the host to promote atherosclerosis, have far greater prospects for success.

miRNA

miRNAs have complementary sequences in the 3' utr and 5' utr of target mRNAs of protein-coding genes, and cause mRNA cleavage or repression of translational machinery. In diseased vacular vessels, miRNAs are dysregulated and highly expressed. miR-33 is found in cardiovascular diseases. It is involved in atherosclerotic initiation and pregression including lipid metabolism, insulin signaling and glucose homeostatis, cell type progression and proliferation, and myeloid cell differentialtion. It was found in rodant that the inhibition of miR-33 will raise HDL level and the expression of miR-33 is down regulated in human with atherosclerotic plaques.

miR-33a and miR-33b are located on intron 16 of human sterol regulatory element-binding protein 2 (SREBP2) gene on chromosome 22 and intron 17 of SREBP1 gene on chromosome 17 miR-33a/b regulates cholesterol/lipid homeostatis by binding in the 3'UTRs of genes involved in cholesterol transport such as ATP binding Cassette (ABC) transporters and enhance or represses its expression. Study have shown that ABCA1 mediates transport of cholesterol from peripheral tissues to Apolupoprotein-1 and it is also important in the reverse cholesterol transport pathway, where cholesterol is deliverd from peripheral tissue to the liver, where it can be excreted into bile or converted to bile acids prior to excretion. Therefore, we know that ABCA1 plays an important role in preventing cholesterol accumulation in macrophages. By enhancing miR-33 function, the level of ABCA1 is decreased, leading to decrease cellular cholesterol efflux to apoA-1. On the other hand, by inhibiting miR-33 function, the level of ABCA1 is increased and increases the cholesterol efflux to apoA-1. Suppression of miR-33 will lead to less cellular cholesterol and higher plasma HDL level through the regulation of ABCA1 expression. [Wikipedia]

Folks, the reason for this, piece is just informational, not to give you bragging rights with your doctor. The definitely know much more and better. If you suspect a need for help in this area, please consult your physician and do not even attempt to self diagnose or medicate. If you do, the risk will be on you, and it may be too much to handle. This entire book is not a medical advice, just a piece of information, to heighten your awareness and also a little insightful understanding. Though not enough to diagnose and treat anything.

Hyperinsulinemia

Hyperinsulinemia is simply a condition whereby there is too much insulin in the blood than practically needed. This often predicates the onset of diabetes. I will again go to Wiki for more insight that we can all share about the phenomena:

"Hyperinsulinemia, or hyperinsulinaemia is a condition in which there are excess levels of insulin circulating in the blood than expected relative to the level of glucose. While it is often mistaken for diabetes or hyperglycaemia, hyperinsulinemia can result from a variety of metabolic diseases and conditions. While hyperinsulinemia is often seen in people with early stage type 2 diabetes mellitus, it is not the cause of the condition and is only one symptom of the disease. Type 2 diabetes only occurs when pancreatic beta-cell function is impaired. Hyperinsulinemia can be seen in a variety of conditions including diabetes mellitus type 2, in neonates and in drug induced hyperinsulinemia. It can also occur in congenital hyperinsulism, including nesidioblastosis. Hyperinsulinemia is associated with hypertension, obesity, dyslipidemia, and glucose intolerance. These conditions are collectively known as Metabolic syndrome. This close association between hyperinsulinemia and conditions of metabolic syndrome suggest related or common mechanisms of pathogenicity. Hyperinsulinemia has been shown to "play a role in obese hypertension by increasing renal sodium retention"

In type 2 diabetes, the cells of the body become resistant to the effects of insulin as the receptors which bind to the hormone become less sensitive to insulin concentrations resulting in hyperinsulinemia and disturbances in insulin release. With a reduced response to insulin, the beta cells of the pancreas secrete increasing amounts of insulin in response to the continued high blood glucose levels resulting in hyperinsulinemia. In insulin resistant tissues, a threshold concentration of insulin is reached causing the cells to uptake glucose and therefore decreases blood glucose levels. Studies have shown that the high levels of insulin resulting from insulin resistance might enhance insulin resistance.

Studies on mice with genetically reduced circulating insulin suggest that hyperinsulinemia plays a causal role in high fat diet-induced obesity. In this study, mice with reduced insulin levels expended more energy and had fat cells that were reprogrammed to burn some energy as heat.

Hyperinsulinemia in neonates can be the result of a variety of environmental and genetic factors. If the mother of the infant is a diabetic, and does not properly control her blood glucose levels, the hyperglycemic maternal blood can create a hyperglycemic environment in the fetus. To compensate for the increased blood glucose levels, fetal pancreatic beta cells can undergo hyperplasia. The rapid division of beta cells results in increased levels of insulin being secreted to compensate for the high blood glucose levels. Following birth, the hyperglycemic maternal blood is no longer accessible to the neonate resulting in a rapid drop in the newborn's blood glucose levels. As insulin levels are still elevated this results in hyperinsulinemia. To treat the condition, high concentration doses of glucose are given to the neonate as required maintaining normal blood glucose levels. The hyperinsulinemia condition subsides after one to two days.

Insulin resistance (IR) is a physiological condition in which cells fail to respond to the normal actions of the hormone insulin. The body produces insulin, but the cells in the body become resistant to insulin and are unable to use it as effectively, leading to hyperglycemia. Beta cells in the pancreas subsequently increase their production of insulin, further contributing to hyperinsulinemia. This often remains undetected and can contribute to a diagnosis of Type 2 Diabetes.

Explanation

One of insulin's functions is to regulate delivery of glucose into cells to provide them with energy. Insulin resistant cells cannot take in glucose, amino acids and fatty acids. Thus, glucose, fatty acids and amino acids 'leak' out of the cells. A decrease in insulin/glucagon ratio inhibits glycolysis which in turn decreases energy production. The resulting increase in blood glucose may raise levels outside the normal range and cause adverse health effects, depending on dietary conditions.

Certain cell types such as fat and muscle cells require insulin to absorb glucose. When these cells fail to respond adequately to circulating insulin, blood glucose levels rise. The liver helps regulate glucose levels by reducing its secretion of glucose in the presence of insulin. This normal reduction in the liver's glucose production may not occur in people with insulin resistance.

Insulin resistance in muscle and fat cells reduces glucose uptake (and also local storage of glucose as glycogen and triglycerides, respectively), whereas insulin resistance in liver cells results in reduced glycogen synthesis and storage and also a failure to suppress glucose production and release into the blood.

Insulin resistance normally refers to reduced glucose-lowering effects of insulin. However, other functions of insulin can also be affected. For example, insulin resistance in fat cells reduces the normal effects of insulin on lipids and results in reduced uptake of circulating lipids and increased hydrolysis of stored triglycerides. Increased mobilization of stored lipids in these cells elevates free fatty acids in the blood plasma. Elevated blood fatty-acid concentrations (associated with insulin resistance and diabetes mellitus Type 2), reduced muscle glucose uptake, and increased liver glucose production all contribute to elevated blood glucose levels. High plasma levels of insulin and glucose due to insulin resistance are a major component of the metabolic syndrome. If insulin resistance exists, more insulin needs to be secreted by the pancreas. If this compensatory increase does not occur, blood glucose concentrations increase and type 2 diabetes occurs.

Signs and symptoms

This section possibly contains original research. Relevant discussion may be found on Talk:Insulin resistance. Please improve it by verifying the claims made and adding inline citations. Statements consisting only of original research may be removed. (October 2010)

These depend on poorly understood variations in individual biology and consequently may not be found with all people diagnosed with insulin resistance. Brain fogginess and inability to focus. High blood sugar.Intestinal bloating – most intestinal gas is produced from carbohydrates in the diet, mostly those that humans cannot digest and absorb.

Weight gain, fat storage, difficulty losing weight – for most people, excess weight is from high fat storage; the fat in IR is generally stored in and around abdominal organs in both males and females. It is currently suspected that hormones produced in that fat are a precipitating cause of insulin resistance.

Increased blood triglyceride levels.

Increased blood pressure. Many people with hypertension are either diabetic or pre-diabetic and have elevated insulin levels due to insulin resistance. One of insulin's effects is to control arterial wall tension throughout the body.

Increased pro-inflammatory cytokines associated with cardiovascular disease.

Depression. Due to the deranged metabolism resulting from insulin resistance, psychological effects, including depression, are not uncommon.

Acanthosis nigricans.

Increased hunger.

Associated Risk Factors

Several associated risk factors include the following:

- Genetic factors (inherited component):
    - family history with type 2 diabetes;
        - Insulin receptor mutations (Donohue Syndrome)
        - LMNA mutations (Familial Partial Lipodystrophy)
        Insulin resistance may also be caused by the damage of liver cells having

    undergone a defect of insulin receptors in hepatocytes.[citation needed]
  - being Black, Hispanic, American Indian or Asian (this is also cultural as diet varies with race and class).

- Particular physiological conditions and environmental factors:
  - being over 40-45 years of age;
  - obesity;
  - one's body storing fat predominantly in the abdomen (also known as "abdominal obesity)", as

opposed to storing it in hips and thighs.
- sedentary lifestyle, lack of physical exercise
- hypertension;
- high triglyceride level (Hypertriglyceridemia);
- low level of high-density lipoprotein (also known as HDL cholesterol or "good cholesterol");pre-diabetes, one's sugar levels in blood have been too high in the past, i.e. one's body has previously shown slight problems with its production and usage of insulin ("previous evidence

of impaired glucose homeostasis");
- having developed gestational diabetes during past pregnancies;
- giving birth to a baby weighing more than 9 pounds (a bit over 4 kilograms)

- Pathology:
  - Obesity and Overweight (BMI > 25);
  - Metabolic syndrome (Hyperlipidemia + HDL cholesterol level <

0.90 mmol/L or triglyceride level > 2.82 mmol/L); Hypertension (> 140/90 mmHg) or arteriosclerosis;
- Liver pathologies;
- Infection (Hepatitis C[7]);
- Haemochromatosis;
- Gastroparesis;
- Polycystic ovary syndrome (PCOS);

Hypercortisolism (e.g., steroid use or Cushing's disease);

Medication (e.g., glucosamine, rifampicin, isoniazid, olanzapine, risperidone, progestogens, corticosteroids, glucocorticoids, methadone, many antiretrovirals).

Causes

Diet:

It is well known that insulin resistance commonly coexists with obesity. However, causal links between insulin resistance, obesity, and dietary factors are complex and controversial. It is possible that one of them arises first, and tends to cause the other; or that insulin resistance and excess body weight might arise independently as a consequence of a third factor, but end up reinforcing each other. Some population groups might be genetically predisposed to one or the other.

Dietary fat has long been implicated as a driver of insulin

resistance. Studies on animals have observed significant insulin resistance in rats after just 3 weeks on a high-fat diet (59% fat, 20% carb.) Large quantities of saturated, monounsaturated, and polyunsaturated (omega-6) fats all appear to be harmful to rats to some degree, compared to large amounts of starch, but saturated fat appears to be the most effective at producing IR. This is partly caused by direct effects of a high-fat diet on blood markers, but, more significantly, ad libitum high-fat diet has the tendency to result in caloric intake that's far in excess of animals' energy needs, resulting in rapid weight gain. In humans, statistical evidence is more equivocal. Being insensitive to insulin is still positively correlated with fat intake, and negatively correlated with dietary fiber intake, but both these factors are also correlated with excess body weight.

The effect of dietary fat is largely or completely overridden if the high-fat diet is modified to contain nontrivial quantities (in excess of 5-10% of total fat intake) of polyunsaturated omega-3 fatty acids. This protective effect is most established with regard to the so-called "marine long-chain omega-3 fatty acids", EPA and DHA, found in fish oil; evidence in favor of other omega-3's, in particular, the most common vegetable-based omega-3 fatty acid, ALA, also exists, but it is more limited; some studies find ALA only effective among people with insufficient long-chain omega-3 intake, and some studies fail to find any effect at all (ALA can be partially converted into EPA and DHA by the human body, but the conversion rate is thought to be 10% or less, depending on diet and gender). The effect is thought to explain relatively low incidence of IR, type 2 diabetes, and obesity in polar foragers such as Alaskan Eskimos consuming their ancestral diet (which is very high in fat, but contains substantial amounts of omega-3). However, it is not strong enough to prevent IR in the typical modern Western diet. Unlike their omega-6 counterparts (which can be cheaply produced from a variety of sources, such as corn and soybeans), major sources of omega-3 fatty acids remain relatively rare and expensive. Consequently, the recommended average intake of omega-3 for adult men in the United States is only 1.6 grams/day, or less than 2% of total fat; the actual average consumption of omega-3 in the United States is around 1.3 grams/day, almost all of it in the form of ALA; EPA and DHA contributed less than 0.1 grams/day.

Elevated levels of free fatty acids and triglycerides in the blood stream and tissues have been found in many studies to contribute to diminished insulin sensitivity. Triglyceride levels are driven by a variety of dietary factors. They are correlated with excess body weight. They tend to rise due to overeating and fall during fat loss. At constant energy intake, triglyceride levels are positively correlated with trans fat intake and strongly inversely correlated with omega-3 intake. High-carbohydrate, low-fat diets were found by many studies to result in elevated triglycerides, in part due to higher production of VLDL from fructose and sucrose, and in part because increased carbohydrate intake tends to displace some omega-3 from the diet.

Several recent authors suggested that the intake of simple sugars, and particularly fructose, is also a factor that contributes to insulin resistance. Fructose is metabolized by the liver into triglycerides, and, as mentioned above, tends to raise their levels in the blood stream. Therefore, it may contribute to insulin resistance through the same mechanisms as the dietary fat. Just like fat, high levels of fructose and/or sucrose induce insulin resistance in rats, and, just like with fat, this insulin resistance is ameliorated by fish oil supplementation. One study observed that a low-fat diet high in simple sugars (but not in complex carbohydrates and starches) significantly stimulates fatty acid synthesis, primarily of the saturated fatty acid palmitate, therefore, paradoxically, resulting in the plasma fatty acid pattern that is similar to that produced by a high-saturated-fat diet It should be pointed out that virtually all evidence of deleterious effects of simple sugars so far is limited to their concentrated formulations and sweetened beverages. In particular, very little is known about effects of simple sugars in whole fruit and vegetables. If anything, epidemiological studies suggest that their high consumption is associated with somewhat lower risk of IR and/or metabolic syndrome.

Yet another proposed mechanism involves the phenomenon known as leptin resistance. Leptin is a hormone that regulates long-term energy balance in many mammals. An important role of leptin is long-term inhibition of appetite in response to formation of body fat. This mechanism is known to be disrupted in many obese individuals: even though their leptin levels are commonly elevated, this does not result in reduction of appetite and caloric intake. Leptin resistance can be triggered in rats by ad libitum consumption of energy-dense, highly palatable foods over a period of several days. Chronic consumption of fructose in rats ultimately results in leptin resistance (however, this has only been demonstrated in a diet where fructose provided 60% of calories; the actual consumption by humans in a typical Western diet is several times lower.) Once leptin signalling has been disrupted, the individual becomes prone to further overeating, weight gain, and insulin resistance.

As elevated blood glucose levels are the primary stimulus for insulin secretion and production, habitually excessive carbohydrate intake is another likely contributor. This serves as a major motivation behind the low-carb family of diets. Furthermore, carbohydrates are not equally absorbed (for example, the blood glucose level response to a fixed quantity of carbohydrates in baked potatoes is about twice the response to the same quantity of carbohydrates in pumpernickel bread). Integrated blood glucose response to a fixed quantity of carbohydrates in a meal is known as glycemic index. Some diets are based on this concept, assuming that consumption of low-GI foods is less likely to result in insulin resistance and obesity. However, small to moderate amounts of simple sugars (i.e., sucrose, fructose, and glucose) in the typical developed-world diet seem to not have a causative effect on the development of insulin resistance.

Once established, insulin resistance would result in increased circulating levels of insulin. Since insulin is the primary hormonal signal for energy storage into fat cells, which tend to retain their sensitivity in the face of hepatic and skeletal muscle resistance, IR stimulates the formation of new fatty tissue and accelerates weight gain.

Another possible explanation is that both insulin resistance and obesity often have the same cause, a systematic overeating, which has the potential to lead to insulin resistance and obesity due to repeated administration of excess levels of glucose, which stimulate insulin secretion; excess levels of fructose, which raise triglyceride levels in the bloodstream; and fats, which can be easily absorbed by the adipose cells and tend to end up as fatty tissue in a hypercaloric diet. Some scholars go as far as to claim that neither insulin resistance, nor obesity are really metabolic disorders per se, but simply adaptive responses to sustained caloric surplus, intended to protect bodily organs from lipotoxicity (unsafe levels of lipids in the bloodstream and tissues): "Obesity should therefore not be regarded as a pathology or disease, but rather as the normal, physiologic response to sustained caloric surplus... As a consequence of the high level of lipid accumulation in insulin target tissues including skeletal muscle and liver, it has been suggested that exclusion of glucose from lipid-laden cells is a compensatory defense against further accumulation of lipogenic substrate." Fast food meals typically possess several characteristics, all of which have independently been linked to IR: they are energy-dense, palatable, and cheap, increasing risk of overeating and leptin resistance; they are simultaneously high in dietary fat and fructose, and low in omega-3; and they usually have high glycemic indices. Consumption of fast food has been proposed as a fundamental factor behind the metabolic syndrome epidemic and all its constituents. An American study has shown that glucosamine (often prescribed for joint problems) may cause insulin resistance.

Studies show that high levels of cortisol within the bloodstream from the digestion of animal protein can contribute to the development of insulin resistance. Additionally, animal protein, because of its high content of purine, causes blood pH to become acidic. Several studies conclude that high uric acid levels, apart from other contributing factors, by itself may be a significant cause of insulin resistance.

Vitamin D deficiency is also associated with insulin resistance.

Sedentary lifestyle

Sedentary lifestyle increases the likelihood of development of insulin resistance. It's been estimated that each

500 kcal/week increment in physical activity related energy expenditure reduces the lifetime risk of type 2 diabetes by 6%. A different study found that vigorous exercise at least once a week reduced the risk of type 2 diabetes in women by 33%.

Protease inhibitors

Protease inhibitors found in HIV drugs are linked to insulin resistance.

Cellular

At the cellular level, much of the variance in insulin sensitivity between untrained, non-diabetic humans can be explained by two mechanisms: differences in phospholipids profiles of skeletal muscle cell membranes, and in intramyocellular lipid (ICML) stores within these cells. High levels of lipids in the bloodstream have the potential to result in accumulation of triglycerides and their derivatives within muscle cells, which activate proteins Kinase C-ε and C-θ, ultimately reducing the glucose uptake at any given level of insulin. This mechanism is quite fast-acting and can induce insulin resistance within days or even hours in response to a large lipid influx. Draining the intracellular reserves, on the other hand, is more challenging: moderate caloric restriction alone, even over a period of several months, appears to be ineffective, and it must be combined with physical exercise to have any effect. However, a 2011 study found that a severe ultra-low-calorie diet, limiting patients to 600 calories/day for a period of 2 months, without explicit exercise targets, was capable of reversing insulin resistance and type 2 diabetes.)

In the long term, diet has the potential to change the ratio of polyunsaturated to saturated phospholipids in cell membranes, correspondingly changing cell membrane fluidity; full impact of such changes is not fully understood, but it is known that the percentage of polyunsaturated phospholipids is strongly inversely correlated with insulin resistance. It is hypothesized that increasing cell membrane fluidity by increasing PUFA concentration might result in an enhanced number of insulin receptors, an increased affinity of insulin to its receptors and a reduced insulin resistance, and vice versa.

Many stressing factors can lead to increased cortisol in the bloodstream. Cortisol counteracts insulin, and contributes to hyperglycemia-causing hepatic gluconeogenesis and inhibits the peripheral utilization of glucose which eventually leads to insulin resistance. It does this by decreasing the translocation of glucose transporters (especially GLUT4) to the cell membrane.

Although inflammation is often caused by cortisol, inflammation by itself also seems to be implicated in causing insulin resistance. Mice without JNKIsignaling do not develop insulin resistance under dietary conditions that normally produce it.

Rare type 2 diabetes cases sometimes use high levels of exogenous insulin. As short term overdosing of insulin causes short term insulin resistance, it has been hypothesized that chronic high dosing contributes to more permanent insulin resistance.[citation needed]

Molecular

Insulin resistance has been proposed at a molecular level to be a reaction to excess nutrition by superoxide dismutase in cell mitochondria that acts as an antioxidant defense mechanism. This link seems to exist under diverse causes of insulin resistance. It is also based on the finding that insulin resistance can be rapidly reversed by exposing cells to mitochondrial uncouplers, electron transport chain inhibitors, or mitochondrial superoxide dismutase mimetics.

Disease

Recent research and experimentation has uncovered a non-obesity related connection to insulin resistance and type 2 diabetes. It has long been observed that patients who have had some kinds of bariatric surgery have increased insulin sensitivity and even remission of type 2 diabetes. It was discovered that diabetic/insulin resistant non obese rats whose duodenum has been surgically removed also experienced increased insulin sensitivity and remission of type 2 diabetes. This suggested similar surgery in humans, and early reports in prominent medical journals (January 8) are that the same effect is seen in humans, at least the small number who have participated in the experimental surgical program. The speculation is that some substance is produced in that portion of the small intestine that signals body cells to become insulin resistant. If the producing tissue is removed, the signal ceases and body cells revert to normal insulin sensitivity. No such substance has been found as yet, so its existence remains speculative.[citation needed]

Insulin resistance has also been linked to PCOS (polycystic ovary syndrome) as either causing it or being caused by it. Further studies are in progress.[citation needed]

HCV and Insulin Resistance

Hepatitis C also makes people three to four times more likely to develop type 2 diabetes and insulin resistance. In addition, "people with Hepatitis C who develop diabetes probably have susceptible insulin-producing cells, and would probably get it anyway – but much later in life The extra insulin resistance caused by Hepatitis C apparently brings on diabetes at 35 or 40, instead of 65 or 70."

Pathophysiology

Any food or drink containing glucose (or the digestible carbohydrates that contain it, such as sucrose, starch, etc.) causes blood glucose levels to increase. In normal metabolism, the elevated blood glucose level instructs beta (β) cells in the Islets of Langerhans, located in the pancreas, to release insulin into the blood. The insulin, in turn, makes insulin-sensitive tissues in the body (primarily skeletal muscle cells, adipose tissue, and liver) absorb glucose, and thereby lower the blood glucose level. The beta cells reduce insulin output as the blood glucose level falls, allowing blood glucose to settle at a constant of approximately 5 mmol/L (mM) (90 mg/dL). In an insulin-resistant person, normal levels of insulin do not have the same effect in controlling blood glucose levels. During the compensated phase on insulin resistance insulin levels are higher, and blood glucose levels are still maintained. If compensatory insulin secretion fails, then either fasting (impaired fasting glucose) or postprandial (impaired glucose tolerance) glucose concentrations increase. Eventually, type 2 diabetes occurs when glucose levels become higher throughout the day as the resistance increases and compensatory insulin secretion fails. The elevated insulin levels also have additional effects (see insulin) that cause further abnormal biological effects throughout the body.[citation needed]

The most common type of insulin resistance is associated with overweight and obesity in a condition known as the metabolic syndrome. Insulin resistance often progresses to full Type 2 diabetes mellitus (T2DM). This is often seen when hyperglycemia develops after a meal, when pancreatic β-cells are unable to produce sufficient insulin to maintain normal blood sugar levels (euglycemia) in the face of insulin resistance. The inability of the β-cells to produce sufficient insulin in a condition of hyperglycemia is what characterizes the transition from insulin resistance to T2DM.[64]

Various disease states make body tissues more resistant to the actions of insulin. Examples include infection (mediated by the cytokine TNFα) and acidosis. Recent research is investigating the roles of adipokines (the cytokines produced by adipose tissue) in insulin resistance. Certain drugs may also be associated with insulin resistance (e.g., glucocorticoids).[citation needed]

Insulin itself leads to a kind of insulin resistance; every time a cell is exposed to insulin, the production of GLUT4 (type four glucose receptors) on the cell's membrane decreases somewhat. In the presence of a higher than usual level of insulin (generally caused by insulin resistance), this down-regulation acts as a kind of positive feedback, increasing the need for insulin. Exercise reverses this process in muscle tissue, but if it is left unchecked, it can contribute to insulin resistance.

Elevated blood levels of glucose — regardless of cause — lead to increased glycation of proteins with changes, only a few of which are understood in any detail, in protein function throughout the body.

Insulin resistance is often found in people with visceral adiposity (i.e., a high degree of fatty tissue within the abdomen — as distinct from subcutaneous adiposity or fat between the skin and the muscle wall, especially elsewhere on the body, such as hips or thighs), hypertension, hyperglycemia and dyslipidemia involving elevated triglycerides, small dense low-density lipoprotein (sdLDL) particles, and decreased HDL cholesterol levels. With respect to visceral adiposity, a great deal of evidence suggests two strong links with insulin resistance. First, unlike subcutaneous adipose tissue, visceral adipose cells produce significant amounts of proinflammatory cytokines such as tumor necrosis factor-alpha (TNF-a), and Interleukins-1 and -6, etc. In numerous experimental models, these proinflammatory cytokines disrupt normal insulin action in fat and muscle cells, and may be a major factor in causing the whole-body insulin resistance observed in patients with visceral adiposity. Much of the attention on production of proinflammatory cytokines has focused on the IKK-beta/NF-kappa-B pathway, a protein network that enhances transcription of inflammatory markers and mediators that can cause insulin resistance. Second, visceral adiposity is related to an accumulation of fat in the liver, a condition known as non-alcoholic fatty liver disease (NAFLD). The result of NAFLD is an excessive release of free fatty acids into the bloodstream (due to increased lipolysis), and an increase in hepatic glycogenolysis and hepatic glucose production, both of which have the effect of exacerbating peripheral insulin resistance and increasing the likelihood of Type 2 diabetes mellitus.[citation needed]

Insulin resistance is also often associated with a hypercoagulable state (impaired fibrinolysis) and increased inflammatory cytokine levels. [Wikipedia]

Adiposity

This section is very well explained by Wiki. Again I will be hands off and just start the quote:

"In biology, adipose tissue or body fat or just fat is loose connective tissue composed mostly of adipocytes. In addition to adipocytes, adipose tissue contains the stromal vascular fraction (SVF) of cells including preadipocytes, fibroblasts, vascular endothelial cells and a variety of immune cells (i.e. adipose tissue macrophages (ATMs)). Adipose tissue is derived from preadipocytes. Its main role is to store energy in the form of lipids, although it also cushions and insulates the body. Far from hormonally inert, adipose tissue has, in recent years, been recognized as a major endocrine organ, as it produces hormones such as leptin, estrogen, resistin, and the cytokine TNFα. Moreover, adipose tissue can affect other organ systems of the body and may lead to disease. Obesity or being overweight in humans and most animals does not depend on body weight, but on the amount of body fat—to be specific, adipose tissue.[citation needed] The two types of adipose tissue are white adipose tissue (WAT) and brown adipose tissue (BAT). The formation of adipose tissue appears to be controlled in part by the adipose gene. Adipose tissue – more specifically brown adipose tissue – was first identified by the Swiss naturalist Conrad Gessner in 1551.

Anatomical features

In humans, adipose tissue is located beneath the skin (subcutaneous fat), around internal organs (visceral fat), in bone marrow (yellow bone marrow) and in the breast tissue. Adipose tissue is found in specific locations, which are referred to as adipose depots. Apart from adipocytes, which comprise the highest percentage of cells within adipose tissue, other cell types are present, collectively termed stromal vascular fraction (SVF) of cells. SVF includes preadipocytes, fibroblasts, adipose tissue macrophages, and endothelial cells. Adipose tissue contains many small blood vessels. In the integumentary system, which includes the skin, it accumulates in the deepest level, the subcutaneous layer, providing insulation from heat and cold. Around organs, it provides protective padding. However, its main function is to be a reserve of lipids, which can be burned to meet the energy needs of the body and to protect it from excess glucose by storing triglycerides produced by the liver from sugars, although some evidence suggests that most lipid synthesis from carbohydrates occurs in the adipose tissue itself. Adipose depots in different parts of the body have different biochemical profiles. Under normal conditions, it provides feedback for hunger and diet to the brain.

Mice have eight major adipose depots, four of which are within the abdominal cavity. The paired gonadal depots are attached to the uterus and ovaries in females and the epididymis and testes in males; the paired retroperitoneal depots are found along the dorsal wall of the abdomen, surrounding the kidney, and, when massive, extend into the pelvis. The mesenteric depot forms a glue-like web that supports the intestines and the omental depot (which originates near the stomach and spleen) and - when massive - extends into the ventral abdomen. Both the mesenteric and omental depots incorporate much lymphoid tissue as lymph nodes and milky spots, respectively. The two superficial depots are the paired inguinal depots, which are found anterior to the upper segment of the hind limbs (underneath the skin) and the subscapular depots, paired medial mixtures of brown adipose tissue adjacent to regions of white adipose tissue, which are found under the skin between the dorsal crests of the scapulae. The layer of brown adipose tissue in this depot is often covered by a "frosting" of white adipose tissue; sometimes these two types of fat (brown and white) are hard to distinguish. The inguinal depots enclose the inguinal group of lymph nodes. Minor depots include the pericardial, which surrounds the heart, and the paired popliteal depots, between the major muscles behind the knees, each containing one large lymph node. Of all the depots in the mouse, the gonadal depots are the largest and the most easily dissected, comprising about 30% of dissectible fat.

Obesity

In an obese person, excess adipose tissue hanging downward from the abdomen is referred to as a panniculus (or pannus). A panniculus complicates surgery of the morbidly obese individual. It may remain as a literal "apron of skin" if a severely obese person quickly loses large amounts of fat (a common result of gastric bypass surgery). This condition cannot be effectively corrected through diet and exercise alone, as the panniculus consists of adipocytes and other supporting cell types shrunken to their minimum volume and diameter.[citation needed] Reconstructive surgery is one method of treatment.

Obesity and cancer

According to the International Agency for Research on Cancer, and based on epidemiological studies, obese or overweight people are at increased risk of developing several cancer types, such as adenocarcinoma of the oesophagus; colon cancer; breast cancer (in postmenopausal women); endometrial cancer; and kidney cancer.

Abdominal fat

Visceral fat or abdominal fat (also known as organ fat or intra-abdominal fat) is located inside the abdominal cavity, packed between the organs (stomach, liver, intestines, kidneys, etc.). Visceral fat is different from subcutaneous fat underneath the skin, and intramuscular fat interspersed in skeletal muscles. Fat in the lower body, as in thighs and buttocks, is subcutaneous and is not consistently spaced tissue, whereas fat in the abdomen is mostly visceral and semi-fluid. Visceral fat is composed of several adipose depots, including mesenteric, epididymal white adipose tissue (EWAT), and perirenal depots. Visceral fat is considered adipose tissue whereas subcutaneous fat is not considered as such.

An excess of visceral fat is known as central obesity, or "belly fat", in which the abdomen protrudes excessively. Excess visceral fat is also linked to type 2 diabetes, insulin resistance, inflammatory diseases, and other obesity-related diseases.

Female sex hormone causes fat to be stored in the buttocks, thighs, and hips in women. Men are more likely to have fat stored in the belly due to sex hormone differences. When women reach menopause and the estrogen produced by the ovaries declines, fat migrates from the buttocks, hips and thighs to the waist; later fat is stored in the abdomen.

High-intensity exercise is one way to effectively reduce total abdominal fat. One study suggests at least 10 MET-hours per week of aerobic exercise is required for visceral fat reduction.

Epicardial fat

Epicardial adipose tissue (EAT) is a particular form of visceral fat deposited around the heart and found to be a metabolically active organ that generates various bioactive molecules, which might significantly affect cardiac function. Marked component differences have been observed in comparing EAT with subcutaneous fat, suggesting a depot specific impact of stored fatty acids on adipocyte function and metabolism.

Most of the remaining nonvisceral fat is found just below the skin in a region called the hypodermis. This subcutaneous fat is not related to many of the classic obesity-related pathologies, such as heart disease, cancer, and stroke, and some evidence even suggests it might be protective. The typically female (or gynecoid) pattern of body fat distribution around the hips, thighs, and buttocks is subcutaneous fat, and therefore poses less of a health risk compared to visceral fat.

Like all other fat organs, subcutaneous fat is an active part of the endocrine system, secreting the hormones leptin and resistin.

The relationship between the subcutaneous adipose layer and total body fat in a person is often modelled by using regression equations. The most popular of these equations was formed by Durnin and Wormersley, who rigorously tested many types of skinfold, and, as a result, created two formulae to calculate the body density of both men and women. These equations present an inverse correlation between skinfolds and body density—as the sum of skinfolds increases, the body density decreases.

Factors such as sex, age, population size or other variables may make the equations invalid and unusable, and, as of 2012, Durnin and Wormersley's equations remain only estimates of a person's true level of fatness. New formulae are still being created.

Ectopic fat

Ectopic fat is fat that is stored in relatively high amounts around the organs of the abdominal cavity, but is not to be confused as visceral fat.

Physiology

Free fatty acids are liberated from lipoproteins by lipoprotein lipase (LPL) and enter the adipocyte, where they are reassembled into triglycerides by esterifying it onto glycerol. Human fat tissue contains about 87% lipids.

There is a constant flux of FFA (Free Fatty Acids) entering and leaving adipose tissue. The net direction of this flux is controlled by insulin and leptin—if insulin is elevated there is a net inward flux of FFA, and only when insulin is low can FFA leave adipose tissue. Insulin secretion is stimulated by high blood sugar, which results from consuming carbohydrates.

In humans, lipolysis (hydrolysis of triglycerides into free fatty acids) is controlled through the balanced control of lipolytic β-adrenergic receptors and α2A-adrenergic receptor-mediated antilipolysis.

Fat cells have an important physiological role in maintaining triglyceride and free fatty acid levels, as well as determining insulin resistance. Abdominal fat has a different metabolic profile—being more prone to induce insulin resistance. This explains to a large degree why central obesity is a marker of impaired glucose tolerance and is an independent risk factor for cardiovascular disease (even in the absence of diabetes mellitus and hypertension). Studies of female monkeys at Wake Forest University (2009) discovered that individuals suffering from higher stress have higher levels of visceral fat in their bodies. This suggests a possible cause-and-effect link between the two, wherein stress promotes the accumulation of visceral fat, which in turn causes hormonal and metabolic changes that contribute to heart disease and other health problems.

Recent advances in biotechnology have allowed for the harvesting of adult stem cells from adipose tissue, allowing stimulation of tissue regrowth using a patient's own cells. In addition, adipose-derived stem cells from both human and animals reportedly can be efficiently reprogrammed into induced pluripotent stem cells without the need for feeder cells.[29] The use of a patient's own cells reduces the chance of tissue rejection and avoids ethical issues associated with the use of human embryonic stem cells.

Adipose tissue is the greatest peripheral source of aromatase in both males and females.[citation needed] contributing to the production of estradiol.

Adipose derived hormones include:

Adiponectin

Resistin

Plasminogen activator inhibitor-1 (PAI-1)

TNFα

IL-6

Leptin

Estradiol (E2)

Adipose tissues also secrete a type of cytokines (cell-to-cell signalling proteins) called adipokines (adipocytokines), which play a role in obesity-associated complications. Perivascular adipose tissue releases adipokines such as adiponectin that affect the contractile function of the vessels that they surround.

Brown fat

A specialized form of adipose tissue in humans, most rodents and small mammals, and some hibernating animals, is brown fat or brown adipose tissue. It is located mainly around the neck and large blood vessels of the thorax. This specialized tissue can generate heat by "uncoupling" the respiratory chain of oxidative phosphorylation within mitochondria. The process of uncoupling means that when protons transit down the electrochemical gradient across the inner mitochondrial membrane, the energy from this process is released as heat rather than being used to generate ATP. This thermogenic process may be vital in neonates exposed to cold, which then require this thermogenesis to keep warm, as they are unable to shiver, or take other actions to keep themselves warm.

Attempts to simulate this process pharmacologically have so far been unsuccessful. Techniques to manipulate the differentiation of "brown fat" could become a mechanism for weight loss therapy in the future, encouraging the growth of tissue with this specialized metabolism without inducing it in other organs.

Until recently, brown adipose tissue was thought to be primarily limited to infants in humans, but new evidence has now overturned that belief. Metabolically active tissue with temperature responses similar to brown adipose was first reported in the neck and trunk of some human adults in 2007, and the presence of brown adipose in human adults was later verified histologically in the same anatomical regions.

Genetics

The thrifty gene hypothesis (also called the famine hypothesis) states that in some populations the body would be more efficient at retaining fat in times of plenty, thereby endowing greater resistance to starvation in times of food scarcity. This hypothesis has been discredited by physical anthropologists, physiologists, and the original proponent of the idea himself.

In 1995, Jeffrey Friedman, in his residency at the Rockefeller University, together with Rudolph Leibel, Douglas Coleman et al. discovered the protein leptin that the genetically obese mouse lacked. Leptin is produced in the white adipose tissue and signals to the hypothalamus. When leptin levels drop, the body interprets this as a loss of energy, and hunger increases. Mice lacking this protein eat until they are four times their normal size.

Leptin, however, plays a different role in diet-induced obesity in rodents and humans. Because adipocytes produce leptin, leptin levels are elevated in the obese. However, hunger remains, and - when leptin levels drop due to weight loss - hunger increases. The drop of leptin is better viewed as a starvation signal than the rise of leptin as a satiety signal. However, elevated leptin in obesity is known as leptin resistance. The changes that occur in the hypothalamus to result in leptin resistance in obesity are currently the focus of obesity research.

Gene defects in the leptin gene (ob) are rare in human obesity. As of July, 2010, only 14 individuals from five families have been identified worldwide who carry a mutated ob gene (one of which was the first ever identified cause of genetic obesity in humans)—two families of

Pakistani origin living in the UK, one family living in Turkey, one in Egypt, and one in Austria—and two other families have been found that carry a mutated ob receptor. Others have been identified as genetically partially deficient in leptin, and, in these individuals, leptin levels on the low end of the normal range can predict obesity.

Several mutations of genes involving the melanocortins (used in brain signaling associated with appetite) and their receptors have also been identified as causing obesity in a larger portion of the population than leptin mutations. In 2007, researchers isolated the adipose gene, which those researchers hypothesize serves to keep animals lean during times of plenty. In that study, increased adipose gene activity was associated with slimmer animals. Although its discoverers dubbed this gene the adipose gene, it is not a gene responsible for creating adipose tissue.

Physical properties

Adipose tissue has a density of ~0.9 g/ml. Thus, a person with more adipose tissue will float more easily than a person of the same weight with more muscular tissue, since muscular tissue has a density of 1.06 g/ml.

Body fat meter

A body fat meter is a widely available tool used to measure the percentage of fat in the human body. Different meters use various methods to determine the body fat to weight ratio. They tend to under-read body fat percentage.

In contrast with clinical tools, one relatively inexpensive type of body fat meter uses the principle of bioelectrical impedance analysis (BIA) in order to determine an individual's body fat percentage. To achieve this, the meter passes a small, harmless, electric current through the body and measures the resistance, then uses information on the person's weight, height, age, and sex to calculate an approximate value for the person's body fat percentage. The calculation measures the total volume of water in the body (lean tissue and muscle contain a higher percentage of water than fat), and estimates the percentage of fat based on this information. The result can fluctuate several percentage points depending on what has been eaten and how much water has been drunk before the analysis. [Wikipedia]

To this end I believe we have all been fairly educated by the Wiki folks regarding the various phenomena explained above. The intent though is to highlight the pathogenesis of metabolic syndrome and it associated indication. I think, if you would agree with me, they did a great job, and also we had a bit more than needed. This section though is just to shed some light on the nuances of the obesity co-morbidities that can complicate one's life, if not that lucky. I will end with a thank you for Wiki again.

Obesity Cost Outcomes

As I mentioned earlier somewhere, obesity and related co-morbidities cost the global community, about 75% of the aggregate, healthcare expenditure. In the United States alone, the cost is approximately $150 Billion, and it is still on an upward swing, if not contained. I am hopeful though that, it will be soon. Let us all give it the sense of urgency warranted. There are other numbers, but I think these are enough for us to judge the magnitude of the impact. Any more will be an over kill.

In addition to the monetary cost to society, the psychosocial impact is also huge. As I have always been saying, the issues relating to obesity definitely transcends ethnic and national boundaries. It may replicate itself differently within varying anthropological nuances of different societies, yet the main core issues are the same. I read a report, written by a lady from Ireland, whose name I will provide shortly.

The report was for a research she did in Ireland, with the intent of understanding the psychosocial impact of obesity on a specified sample from a population in Ireland. I did a brief summary of the report, highlighting the salient point.

Though, I have never been to Ireland, and the closest I have been is England. The facts and finding expressed really resonated with some observations I have made or even read about in some medical literature, specifying different population sample from other parts of the world. I say this to say simply that, it is a humanity issue, which permeates all cultures, though some have done a little better in its containment.

The following summarizes the main issues discussed in the report, though not in its entirety:

MAIN THESIS:

The Psychological Aspects of Obesity: A qualitative and Quantitative Study. (By Mary Rosaleen Cawley, Department of General Practice and Primary Care [Division of Community Based Sciences] University of Glasgow (October 2004)

The Psychological Aspects of Obesity

Main Goal of the Research Study and Questions:

> ➢ The Health Services Research (PhD), funded by the Chief Scientist Office (CSO), investigated the psychosocial aspects of Obesity in the community sample of men, and women aged 30 – 60, Living in deprived, and affluent areas of Greater Glasgow area.

Specific Objectives of the Study

➤ To determine the relationship between Obesity and Psychosocial health (taking into account body satisfaction and self-esteem), and investigate whether the relationship between obesity and psychosocial health is similar or different for men and women.

➤ To explore participants knowledge about the causes of obesity.

➤ To explore the mechanisms through which weight and

psychological health are linked using semi-structured interviews.

Method

> The Study incorporated a mixed method design, and combined a community-health survey, and semi-structured interviews with a purposively selected sub-sample of questionnaire respondents. 52% of participants who completed the questionnaire were obese or

overweight and 16% were defined as obese.

➢ Obesity and body image were not significant predictors of poor psychological health. Furthermore, low self-esteem was the most significant predictor of poor psychological health for both men and women.

➢ Results:

➢ The quantitative and qualitative findings demonstrated that the obese individuals are aware of their current weight status, and express a desire to lose weight. Potential motivating factors for weight loss included health concerns, appearance, and special occasions. Psychological factors such as, increased self-esteem and self confidence were also stated by participants as motivating factors.

Issues

➢ Participants identified issues, or a number of barriers, which prevented them from fully implementing health promotion advice.

➢ Qualitative findings suggested the possibility of cyclical relationship between dieting, depression and emotional eating.

➢ Weight cycling was also observed. (Loosing and regaining weight)

Findings and Conclusions:

➢ Obesity and Psychosocial Health

- Low self-esteem was the most significant predictor of poor psychological health for both men and women.
- The bi-variate co-relational analysis demonstrated a significantly positive association between self-esteem and the MHI -5 scores (A body image measure)
- The qualitative findings highlight that the

mechanisms which links obesity and psychological health are complex.

- 98.5% of obese surveyed participants perceived themselves as obese, and 98% wanted to weigh less, however the men were more satisfied and happier with their weight than the women.

➢ The participants were knowledgeable about obesity, but

perceived the etiology of obesity to be complex. They however attributed it mostly to over eating, sedentary lifestyle, genetics and slow metabolism.

➢ They bought into the promotion of healthy eating and physical activity, however expressed concerns about some barriers that prevent them from achieving such ideal goals.

    a) Availability problem
    b) Accessibility of healthy food

c) Cost
d) Lack of time
e) Family responsibilities
f) Cost of structured exercise
g) Lack of facilities for walking and cycling and also weather deterrents.
h) Cost of maintaining bicycles and Exercise equipments

i) Psychological factors such as obese women being uncomfortable to overexpose themselves in the gym or swimming pool to avoid embarrassments.
j) Experience of weight change and dieting
k) 86.7 % of obese participants

reported that they have previously tried to diet. (e.g. slimming pills, "Fad" diet, sliming clubs. Etc)

l) Obese and morbidly obese interviewers were aware of the physical and psychological benefits of losing weight. (e.g. appearance, special occasions "Weddings"), and psychosocial factors such as increased self-esteem and self-confidence. They are also aware of perceived health benefits.

2. They also reveled that weight cycling: - Loosing and regaining weight was a common experience.

Strengths and Limitations of the Study:

Strengths:

- It makes a contribution to the evidence base about the links between obesity and psychosocial health

- The mixed methodology design was capable of addressing a wide range of questions through the use of the community study and semi-structured interviews.
- The two methods complemented each other and the qualitative and quantitative findings reinforce each other to strengthen the comprehensiveness of the study.
- The use of established and evaluated measures used in the study enabled its findings to be

compared and discussed with reference to previous research.

➢ Being conducted as part of a health services research studentship allowed a wide range of disciplines to be drawn upon. It hence synthesized, medical, epidemiological, psychological and sociological research, providing a more comprehensive picture of the psychological aspects of obesity.

Limitations

➢ The responds rate was respectably (42%) for a community health survey, yet data about weight and psychological health of non-respondents were not available.

➢ Depressed respondents may not have been motivated to complete the questionnaire.

➢ Higher rate of response sent could have yielded better findings about the psychosocial aspect of obesity.

- Although a cross-sectional study can highlight an association between obesity and psychological health, it cannot illuminate causal pathways as it can only be achieved by using prospective studies.
- Due to the general poor health reputation of Western Scotland, the finding might not be transferable to the general population living outside of the region.

- The computerized system used for the research did not have up to date information about BMI.
- The questionnaire was sent to all patients aged 30 – 60, registered at the practice, rather than solely to obese patients.

Implications to Healthcare professionals

- Participants used terms such as metabolism, genetics to explain the cause of their obesity problem.

- Most patients' attribute the cause of their obesity to: gland/hormone problem, slow metabolism and stress.
- Most general practitioners were more likely to blame obesity on over eating, and sedentary behavior, hence view obesity as a behavior issue.
- Healthcare professionals have tended to use diet and exercise interventions to treat obesity even thought the evidence base about

the most effective intervention is inconclusive.

➢ Most general practitioners believe that they do not have time to treat obesity and do not feel that it is a priority role for them. They believe they have little influence on weight management, hence avoid discussing the subject during consultation.

➢ 19 out of 20 patients acknowledge that they were overweight and were aware of some of the health risks associated with being overweight; hence they avoid using the term obese and fatness. They see them as negative descriptors.

➢ They prefer the terms such as weight, excess weight and BMI. Hence medical professionals should avoid negative descriptors.

➢ In spite of lack of evidence to support the effectiveness of weight loss interventions, weight management groups delivered in primary care, has been fairly effective.

➢ Using a group intervention to targeted obese people with CHD risk factors such as hypertension, type II diabetes and family history of heart disease resulted in significant weight loss, improvement in CHD risk factors and psychological well-being in a three month period

➢ Montage et al (2000) found that although 80% or more of obese participants had received advice, less than 40% had received written material, and less than 20% have visited a nutritionist. Montage et al suggested that oral advice during an appointment will have little impact, and at least some written recommendations will be warranted.

➢ Structured interview that combine nutritional education, and behavioral strategies, and also provide peer support, and group intervention could be offered in primary care as an option for obesity management.

➢ The main role of the GP is to identify suitable patients for the weight management intervention and refer them to a practice nurse, who has been shown to be more motivated to work with obese patients (Mercer & Tessier 2001). The practice nurse should have received structured training on a number of topics, including patient screening and assessment, principles of healthy eating, dietary approaches to weight management, physical activity guide- lines, behavior change strategies and patients monitoring.

➢ Implementing a structured model for weight management is both feasible and effective in primary care (Gibb et al, 2004).

➢ Participants had negative experiences with their GPs, and felt that they regarded all their medical problems to be caused by their weight. As a result they often delay or avoid medical consultation.

➢ The general perception of patients is that, doctors do not do much to help them.

➢ Unsuccessful dieting and failure to maintain weight was a common experience for participants.

➢ Because of problems due to weight cycling, it will be better to encourage people to maintain a stable weight, and improve health by refocusing the issue on fitness, rather than fatness.

➤ Miller & Jacob (2001) argued that diet and exercise interventions are ineffective and are contributing to the prevalence of obesity. Their alternative proposal was "health at any size paradigm ".

➤ Non diet approach has helped obese individuals. (Miller et al 1993). Healthy eating and excersice interventions were found to be more effective.

- Blair et al conducted a prospective study and evaluated the relationship between physical fitness and mortality in men. It was found that unfit men at baseline, with increased level of fitness, reduced their mortality risk by 44%.
- Erlichman, Kerby and James (2002) argued that there is robust evidence to show that physical activity, when considered independently of other factors, is

an important preventive measure for avoiding weight gain.

➢ Ross & Katzmarzy (2003) demonstrated that physical activity reduces abnormal obesity which is strongly associated with type II diabetes and CHD. In addition exercise can also help reduce depression and improve mood, self-esteem, perceptions and quality of life. (Fox, 1999, Paluska and Schweenk 2000)

- Lastly any community program to help in the management of obesity and related health risks should take into consideration all the barriers that prevented patients to effectively implement weight management recommendations.

Implications for Health Promotions

- Participants have absorbed and understand the health promotion message regarding healthy eating.

- Fuller et al (2003) argue that there is a need to acknowledge that patients are not homogeneous passive recipient of information about diet and healthy eating.
- Van Dillen et al (2004) found that overweight people wanted more information about how to lose weight.
- Information needs to be tailored to the needs of obese patients not, "one size fits all".

- Over exposure to health promotion messages can be counterproductive.

  (Van Dillen et al – 2004)

- Fuller et al (2004) heightens that, attempting to change health behavior in Scotland using mass media may not be successful, as participant complain about over exposure and inconsistencies and contradictions in expert advice being given.

- Yen & Syme (1999) suggested that community interventions such as food co-operatives would improve access and availability of fresh vegetables and fruits.
- Horgen & Brownell (2002) compared price change and health message interventions in a delicatessens-style, and found out that price decrease, significantly increased sales of health food. They suggested that, subsidies on healthy food may encourage

consumers to experiment with food choices and buy healthy food.

➢ Prentice and Jebb (2003) suggested amongst others that, fast food vendors could implement healthy eating strategies to help prevent obesity.

➢ Suggested strategies:
  o Providing & promoting a wider range of healthy options.
  o Reducing clear nutritional information.

- - Stop producing "supper sizing".
  - Reducing the amount of fat in food.

Implications of Future Research

- The finding highlights the complexity of the relationship between obesity and psychological health.
  - Recommend the use of prospective studies to further investigate the

causal pathway to obesity and depression.

Other recommendations

- Further research in needed to address the effectiveness of treatment interventions.
- Investigate Long-Term effectiveness of low calories diets.
- Investigate the effectiveness of self management or self help interventions.

- Randomize therapy combined with diet and physical activity in primary care setting.
- Systematic review about the consequences of weight cycling should be conducted.
- Prospective and longitudinal studies, investigating the psychological consequences of weight cycling and dieting should be conducted.

After reading the report, I was quite impress with the authors level of detail and meticulously articulated thought and finding regarding the psychosocial effect of obesity. If you care to learn more, I believe there may be a lot of material on the subject but would recommend that it can be a very good start which will shed a lot of insight to you on the subject. I will thank Mary for sharing his great work to the public. There were really a lot of excellent thought provoking insights. Thanks again.

Equally impressive was a research work done my colleague at Rutgers University, though he was my senior, and graduated even before I entered the program. His work was mainly concerned with cost projections and potential for escalating if current trends are not curtailed. I will also present a short summary of his work:

Modeling and Simulation of Obesity and Related Co-morbidities for Predicting Healthcare Costs. (By Jeffery V. Vernice, Department of Health Informatics. Rutgers Biomedical Sciences – SHRP (July 31, 2007)

Main Goal of Research and Question

The main goal and objectives of the research was to produce a predictive model, demonstrating the impact of obesity nationwide into the next several years.

Special Benefit

The results can help the Healthcare community to address the reduction of obesity complications and co-morbidities in specific segments of the population with different demographic profiles, and ultimately improve the life style of patients and associated cost of related care.

Questions that were addressed

- What is the cost of obesity to the health care providers?

- What factors influence the cost of Obesity

- Are there differences in the cost of care for obesity by state or other socio-economic factors?

- What is the profile of an obese person, and has it changed over time?

- Who will most likely become obese?

- What trend emerged for obese amongst race, age, gender for different co-morbidities?

- What are the differences amongst race, age, gender

or social economic status related to high tech hospital procedures related to obesity

a) What are the differences amongst race age and gender, or social economic status for co-morbidities in the top fifteen causes of death?
b) How do lifestyle choices impact the cost of obesity?

Main Objective of Study

c) To compare the aspects of obesity and co-morbidities, which with others, could influence hospitals' total charges for the obese population, and compare demographic information between the obese and non-obese population. The healthcare cost and utilization project (HCUP) National Impatient Sample (NIS), years (2001 – 2003) data was used.

Method

d) The clinical classified software (CCS) multiple regression tool was used to separate the obese records, using the level 3 label of "Obesity".

e) Two sample t-tests were run for average changes, average age, length of stay, number of diagnosis, and number of procedures for an obese person versus the non-obese person.

f) Comparisons for patients, hospital demographics, and top disease conditions, based on the ICD-9-CM codes were done for the obese versus non person.

g) Factor Analysis was performed in SPSS. Multiple regressions with R^2 in SAS 8.2 were also used.

h) Monte Carlo simulations were then run for the factors most prominent as a result of the multiple regression models.

Results

Total of 176,549 obese records and 4,480,339 non-obese records were extracted for the years 2001 - 2003 for use in the study. The obese population had higher average total changes, ($p < 0.05$) younger average age for a hospital stay and death. ($p < 0.05$), longer length of stay ($p<0.05$), more diagnosis and procedures on average ($p<0.05$) than the non obese population. Several models were the results of multiple regressions based on total changes.

i) The Monte Carlo simulation for normal, uniform and Poisson resulted in some very accurate simulations for specific data elements while others were very inaccurate.

Conclusions

Over all, the obese population has higher total charges on average for all hospital stays and some specific diseases and conditions. Total charges have risen for the obese population from 2001 – 2003. The obese also have a shorter life expectation if death occurs, but have a higher overall death rate. While different models have been developed to determine what factors influence obesity total charges, there are probably other factors which are not included in the NIS. Factors influencing total charges vary depending on the situation. Jeffery, I will also say thank you for the good work.

Though I promised to be simple in my explanations, these caveats are just to give a little more insight to those it might interest. It is ok, if they do not interest you, after all that is not your field of expertise, and you really do not need to know it in great details. However, some people may be interested, and as a result, let us just be fair.

I also believe the humor I throw in here and there, helped got you this far, without being too board. I know otherwise if could have been quite dry to go through this volume so uptight, or worrisome risks obesities posses, especially if you happen to be risk prone to them. Do not lose heart though; you can still do a whole lot to turn things around.

The Pathogenesis of Metabolic Syndrome in Children Lead by Obesity related Issues

I will start this section with two jokes. I hope that will get us off a good start. I also hope it will drive in its main mantra, which though may be hidden in the laughter or smile, it will still come out. Or I will try and do so eventually.

The first joke:

"This though was from Rev. Joel Osteen. He often starts his sermons with jokes, if you are familiar with Rev. Osteen's style.

One thing also that I have observed from him, nothing seems to upset him. In this particular joke, he said, though not verbatim, that: We often blame everyone else about our problems. Especially regarding our body size and eating habits. He then said the problem is not in our stars, but our taste buds! "

I will stop this one here and go to the next one. For that one, I will wind a bit as usual with my jokes before I come to it. As I said earlier, though not perfect, I pride myself for being a Christian. One thing I like most about it, is grace and forgiveness, as it relates to our quest for love and goodness. This has be hammered enough by Rev. Demola and others, and I think it is stuck now.

This may have to do with God's love for me, which also make me want to do just a little to show appreciation. After I learnt how the modulation of "cortisol" the stress hormone that if not well controlled as mentioned before, can cause a lot of harm to you, I realize that God, intentions for all those, was for our own good.

The reason being that, I will caution never to air on the side of rage, either from a traffic jams or anything that may cause some level of irritation, enough to get you on the way to the level of unhealthy excitements. Just trust God and Do just that. That is, if you believe. A flower in a vase or at the garden eventually will die. However, the ones that celebrate love and goodness, like the ROSES, are always remembered. It may be easier said than done, but if you believe as I have said again, it may not be done with your strength. To be fair to others who may not believe in Christianity, there may be mechanisms of similar nature out there. But with me, this works just fine.

I will end this here and go to the next joke. Though I say, I am a Methodist; I am, only because I started that way. I must confess, I got hooked by the music forms they have there. Joining the choir at a very early age, as far back as elementary school, I grew up with hymns. Some classical music from great composers such as Bach, Handel and so on, especially their church compositions, also excited my interest, though just in the enjoyment part. Besides singing I cannot even play a drum. The canticles and the rest also got me hooked.

As loyal as I have been to the Methodist church, I am most loyal to God, though not perfectly. I also had the opportunity to worship elsewhere the word is preached. It is all the same, except the specific cultural nuances. For instance, when I go to the Charismatic Church, I enjoy is as much, though my stiff shy self from my up-bring sometimes just let me ham through their gorgeous rhythms just tapping my feet here and there, without getting on the dance floor. Sometimes I also sing, especially those that I am familiar with.

The bottom line though, is the liturgy, which when grounded in the OLD-OLD story, is the same anywhere. I also had the opportunity to be part of a Catholic Institution. That as I said before, was through my high school days.

My high school was a Catholic Boarding School, a great school which I am very much proud of, in addition to all my Alma Matas. I am because they all contributed to helping me be the way I am today. I watch all kinds of church programs, including the catholic EWTN, TBN and so on. There is a station which is broadcasted from Long Island NY, that I stumbled into one day. It was quite early in the morning, and the program was hosted by Archbishop Fulton Sheen. I would not have enough words to describe his depth of knowledge, on issues he touches on. Though the entire preachers I listen to are equally wonderful in their own styles,

Archbishop Sheen's program that day was stunning yet, with a lot of humor.

If I through in a couple of humor here and there, may be when I grow up I would like to be that funny yet insightful, like Rev. Joel, and Archbishop Sheen, in my own chosen career though may be different at least as I write. Who knows tomorrow?

It may be a bit long and winding up to this point as I already warned you, I trust the joke and it mantra will be well worth it.

Now the Joke:

"Though not verbatim, he said, there was a little boy who lived with his grandma, who has thought him a lot of Christian values. The boy was also very faithful to God. He went out one day, and saw something bad, though he did not intend to. He said it made him feel really bad and guilty. He said the wind blew and unfortunately he saw a lady's underwear.

Disappointed as he was, upon return from town, he rushed to the Grandma and said, I would like to share something I saw whiles in town with you.

She then said what is it? The boy was very disappointed because of what he saw.

After explaining that to the grandma, he asked a few questions. The first one was: did you have anything to do with the wind blowing? The boy said no. Then he asked again, did you pray that the wind blow again? Then he said no again. The last question was, did you follow the girl to the next block? Again he said no. The grandma then finally said, you have nothing to worry about, because you did not sin." I hope this joke was worth the wait.

At this point let's get to business, Childhood Obesity and related problems. Again this is not a religious book per say, yet the principle in the examples being used are quite universal principles. I will therefore try this last one.

Genesis is the first book in the Bible. The first few words that it starts with, says; "In the beginning was the word and the word was with God". Genesis describes what we Christians believe was the beginning of creation and life. The synergy in this discussion is that we are coming to describe the Pathogenesis of metabolic syndrome in children. The word Genesis signifies in both cases the beginning. In children, how life of men starts, genesis synonymously signifies the beginning of life for humans. As again we believe, both the "word" and "God" saves. So does mother and father in the case of a child. However, in the garden there was someone else creeping in to steel their joy. As we know from the story of Adam and Eve, it was the serpent.

In the case of the Child, as it relates to our discussion, the synergy I would like to draw is the role of metabolic syndrome as it relates to the joy and happiness of Children now and in the future. You do not have to be a Christian to appreciate at least the nuances of obesity and metabolic syndrome as it relates to children and their future. We already know the Pathogenesis of metabolic syndrome from the last section, as beautifully explained by our friends in Wiki. By the way, they are a nonprofit, so when they bring their bowl around for collection, please drop in a dime or two.

I am not going to go over it again. There are only two simple points that I will like to make here. Though I have touched on them earlier on, I will reiterate briefly here as well. As I said earlier, women are the bearers of life, as well as its nurturers. At least that was what my mother was for me. If I add prayer warrior, some of you may be mad, though she was also, and I hope you may pardon me. Not that men cannot nurture kids as well, we cannot contend with the woman position as a bearer of life. They are just designed that way.

Usually both parents' genetic compositions and predispositions get hybridized during conception to form the baby. I do not want to waste your time on how chromosomes and other carriers of the human genome is paired and hybridized during conception. "Expensive' went that far, but I still will not go into it. He can be mad all he wants. I still will make Mr. Owusu Mensah proud, and wish this was as physics topic. This book is not a biology book per say and the scope of the topic is not domain appropriate, yet I hope you get my point.

This is not to discount the role men play in the process, though not only the fun part, but also the makeup of the child genetically. Their role is equally important in that regard. As we often have multiple influencing factors triggers a phenomenon, all I am saying here is that, regarding the child's weight, as I have already explained, the women's role is the most dominant one. The child's birth weight is proportional to his mother's birth weight somehow. Also adiposity starts in the womb. A lot of related issues that follows from there have a lot to do with the mother, regarding the child's propensity to be OBESE. I am not saying that is the only influencing factor, yet between the father and the mother, the mother's health, both pre and post natal are very critical to the child's health and well being in general. Of course, relating to the Pathogenesis of metabolic syndrome, just like the serpent, will ultimately steel the ultimate joy of the children, as in the case of Adam and Eve and the rest of the family.

You do not have to believe in the story. But believe it or not, metabolic syndrome is real, even in children and need to be curbed very early. Else, it will be very expensive, not that "Expensive" my biology teacher, to cure its maladies one day, not to talk about their own related miseries and extended burdens on society in general. Many solution works with time, and sometimes, a very long time.

Just like any sound investment planning strategy works very well depending of the longevity of your time horizon. The earlier is always the better, and it is even more so, with investments in our health. If any, I think that is where the thrust should be, though not forgetting also those who are already victims to this situation. If we start early enough, I believe we may have enough saved to probably, spend a little of our wealth in Cancun, or Jamaica, or even Africa and elsewhere we have some good-fun.

The worse part for these kids, even when they get to their teenage years, when they somehow genetically gain superiority over their parents, as they think, though they still need milk, the lack of parental supervision which sometime emanates from socio-cultural and socio-economic nuances of our society, makes the kids really miss out in a lot of ways.

Most of which are detrimental to their future well being as well as even sometimes today's. This much is all I will say at this point. This may end our discussions regarding the pathogenesis of metabolic syndrome in children as they relate to their future.

This is not to get our friends and children in that cohort mad, we all knew better than our parent then, yet they still had relatively more time leverage to drill some stuff in our head. I hope this will make you rather laugh, yet if no one is home to drill much in for you, do it yourself. Reason being that, some of these words of wisdom and knowledge are in books, most of which can be found in libraries all over the place. Have the usual fun, because we also did, yet balance it well with reading.

I promised earlier, that I will shed more light on the two jokes I shared with you:

From Rev. Joel's joke, I would say the gem in it is an advice to develop the taste for the right food groups and simply those that will not adversely affect our health. Archbishop Sheen's joke makes me a bit jealous, and I believe all men should. The reason being that, women have so much power. Only men who want to lie and appear "macho" will disagree with me. In the debate for obesity and its prevention and all, I would like to pose a question. Who has the most power to dictate what men should look, if that look is what they want? I would like all the macho men to keep their answer to themselves. However if you all want to keep it honest, you will agree with me that we will all shape our looks to suite our female partners. This is even more so in the teenage years, as well as courting.

I do not want to through in any long and winding high school stories, though they could have spark some laughter. But I will simply say, if they gung up and dictate a slim look, I bet it will be a fashion statement for all men of all ages for a very long time, saving us money and good health even to enjoy our mutual partnerships and friendships in a clean healthy way. The caveat though is that, they should also live what they preach, or dictates, even if not perfectly.

At least we will understand and match it or even do more to impress! The whole world will be a better place if we all adapt that attitude and style.

The last joke to end this section:

A High school kid once went to his Dad, and said; Daddy, I am easily destructed in school. The Dad said quickly why? Then he said, I would rather ask you a question than explain why. The Dad said, what is your question then? The kid said, at what age, can you willfully keep your eyes of beautiful girls. The Dad took a pulse, yet could not answer the question. He then turned to his 100 year old Dad who lived with them. He then turned back to his son, and said I think Grandpa is older and wiser and can help you better.

He then went to Grandpa, and told his story, with zeal of having the best possible solution to his ordeal in school. The 100 year old grandpa looked at him, and said; son, this is a tough one, you have to ask someone older than me.

SECTION II

Introduction

"The creative systemic integrative thinking approach to problem solving and its application to healthcare and Obesity prevention and management."

Usually in most of my writings, I identify myself as a capitalist. I do so, not to make friends or enemies, but to stand clear of my inclination when it comes to my economics philosophical biases. This though, is not to trash, anybody's philosophical inclination and biases when it comes to economics. The spectrum is quite broad, but leaning toward free market capitalism is the most efficient way of managing our ends.

This though is true, our human weaknesses sometimes gets out of the way, which warrants the need for proper governance and surveillance of certain economic activities, not only to ensure ethical and legal conduct by all players, but to also ensure fairness, and give way to the natural dynamics of the market forces to play out, hence the need for governmental oversight.

Within the spectrum, there are many variations depending on adaptation strategies, given environmental, socio-cultural as well as geo-political nuances and structures already in place to make it work within the natural setting of the adapting country. At the far end, it has been proven by history that, it could lead to economic anarchy upon adherence of its extremities.

The following is a short quote from Wikipedia describing Adams Smith's work in the late 18th century. I quote: "An Inquiry into the Nature and Causes of the Wealth of Nations, generally referred to by its shortened title The Wealth of Nations, is the magnum opus of the Scottish economist and moral philosopher Adam Smith. First published in 1776, the book offers one of the world's first collected descriptions of what builds nations' wealth and is today a fundamental work in classical economics. Through reflection over the economics at the beginning of the Industrial Revolution the book touches upon such broad topics as the division of labor, productivity and free markets".

It is clear from the above quote that, though Adam Smith's work and ideas, at least most of them are still relevant today in classical economics as stated above. Mr. Smith's era, however was at the onset of the industrial revolution, when efficiency and productivity was almost strictly contingent on how well one knows a task and how fast they can work and effectively produce whatever asked to. Work flow efficiency and productivity for more complex products like the auto mobile was measured by how well employees could produce simple tasked very well, and leave it to the next person to complete his own task, that he has mastered so well.

With time, knowledge work and services crept in, with some variances to work flow and division of labor as we knew. The need to collaborate with others to define and deliver, abstract and intangible services became part of our economic activities, a very important part.

This required collaborative efforts with teams some of whom may be doing something completely different from ours, yet every ones piece of work needed to be well meshed, and properly integrated into a coherent document or intellectual property that may have a wealth of value, depending on its purpose, and especially the need it serves its customers.

Such services as Banking and Insurance, Consulting, Healthcare and Manufacturing became so complex that, most companies contracted out nonessential activities and supplies to external vendor, some of whom are local and others international, fueling the complexities of supply chain management issues, relating to such activities.

As the internet evolved with its requisite technological advancements, the complexities of the nuances of the supply and demand model of Economics became so intricately complex. The internet and information technology has eroded many boundaries and demystified many clouds.

The current phenomena of globalization sometimes is even scary, thinking about or just observing from the sidelines the accelerated pace of its dynamics, and the fragile sensitivity to each other's strengths and weaknesses.

The freedom for one to act irrationally on an issue because of claims to national sovereignty is practically illusive in today's global economic arena. In fact we are each other's keeper. As a joke, a sneeze by our great economist, Dr. Alan Greenspan in New York City was heard all over the world. I do not know, how laud, Dr. Greenspan talks, not to even measure his sneeze. Likewise, that of a contemporary in a relatively small but influential sovereign nation like Mexico can have its own ripples that can stretch beyond its boundaries, even if not that far. As we observed earlier in the deprecations of its PASO, and the apparent ripples it caused in the related global financial markets.

At this point, one may be a little agitated, and question the relevance of all this. After all, this is not relevant to economics. What has Obesity got to do with this entire apparently unrelated topic? I will say though that, it has everything to do with it. Though Obesity has some genetic and environment causal factors, it is also largely affected by nutritional consumables and life style choices, which in turn influences our interaction with the related consumer markets.

Our decisions and choices, regarding dietary consumable and lifestyle activities, do not only depend on affordability, though wealth gives us more flexibility and freedom regarding our choices. To many they are restricted by option in the market places of close proximity or at convenient distances.

Though the internet makes distance a bit irrelevant, the speed of delivery depending on needs and the nature of product, makes the good old fashion brick and mortar stores, still maintains reasonable foot traffic. In order words, Obesity is greatly affected by needed solutions and products in the market place, in addition to other factors as already stated.

If any nation prioritizes a healthy population as a major goal, then viewing the nation as a one system, with all its intricate workings gravitating toward that goal, such as a healthy and happy population, interactively with the appropriate collective synergistic team effort, is what will do it. If not, the various sub system, working at their best and with their best efforts only could create anticipated and unanticipated problems for the others.

For instance if unhealthy food is the most available options out there, they may create a great business for fitness centers and other health related businesses, but what will be the overall effective effort of maintenance of good healthy population. I have nothing against the food industry as I have said before, but all I am saying is that, all industries in a particular ecosystem, be it, healthcare or Automotive, should gravitate towards, a common systemic goal. This is often very difficult to achieve, because of the apparent diversity of interests and motivations of the various subsystems. In spite of all of these challenges, a near perfect, or a harmonized solution with a common understanding can better improve the odd of achieving the systemic goals, than the best effort of isolated subsystems.

Hence a creative systemic integrative thinking approach to solving problems being, or potentially being a catalyst to achieving our quest to reaching a harmonized solution, which may not be the ideal solution, but close to it.

Iteratively, with the creative collaboration of all stakeholders, and a commitment to a global systemic goal, a harmonized solution could be reached and improved over time, with dedicated focus on the set goals. For example, if a healthy overall population is the main goal of any sovereign nation as said before, or even the global community, then the theme should permeate and replicate its self in all aspects of socio-economic, socio-cultural and geo-political activities of the people. As I said earlier on, when I first introduced the subject, it may be easier said than done, yet can be done.

With this brief introduction, we may end volume one of this series. As to how the concept is applied in healthcare, especially preventing and managing obesity and related co-morbidities, the concept will be expanded further in volume two of this series. I promised further expansion of some concepts and adverse health risk factors earlier on. This however, will be also in volume two. [Thanks]

www.ingramcontent.com/pod-product-compliance
Lightning Source LLC
Chambersburg PA
CBHW020722180526
45163CB00001B/74